GERMAN
CANCER
THERAPIES

GERMAN

CANCER

THERAPIES

Natural and Conventional Medicines That Offer Hope and Healing

DR. MORTON WALKER

TWIN STREAMS
KENSINGTON PUBLISHING CORP.
http://www.kensingtonbooks.com

This book presents information based upon the research and personal experiences of the author. It is not intended to be a substitute for a professional consultation with a physician or other health-care provider. Neither the publisher nor the author can be held responsible for any adverse effects or consequences resulting from the use of any of the information in this book. They also cannot be held responsible for any errors or omissions in the book. If you have a condition that requires medical advice, the publisher and author urge you to consult a competent health-care professional.

TWIN STREAMS BOOKS are published by

Kensington Publishing Corp.
850 Third Avenue
New York, NY 10022

Copyright © 2003 by Dr. Morton Walker

The list of physicians who practice complementary and alternative medicine in Appendix B is reprinted with permission from the American College for Advancement in Medicine (ACAM).

All Kensington titles, imprints and distributed lines are available at special quantity discounts for bulk purchases for sales promotion, premiums, fund-raising, educational or institutional use.

Special book excerpts or customized printings can also be created to fit specific needs. For details, write or phone the office of the Kensington Special Sales Manager: Kensington Publishing Corp., 850 Third Avenue, New York, NY 10022. Attn. Special Sales Department. Phone: 1-800-221-2647.

Twin Streams and the TS logo Reg. U.S. Pat. & TM Off.

ISBN 1-57566-610-3

First Trade Printing: July 2003
10 9 8 7 6 5 4 3 2 1

Printed in the United States of America

Dedicated to my wife, Joan Walker,
who lost her battle with
inflammatory breast carcinoma

CONTENTS

FOREWORD

Morton Walker, D.P.M. (Doctor of Podiatric Medicine), the author of this book, is my father. Late in 1969 he permanently discontinued the practice of foot surgery in order to utilize his writing skills and become a full-time, freelance medical journalist. For over 33 years he has specialized in researching and writing about holistic medicine, orthomolecular nutrition, and complementary and alternative medicine (CAM). My dad's ultimate goal is the advancement of CAM methods into routine medical practice procedures so that every North American patient has access to them. His special interest is cancer because my mother, Joan Walker, his wife of forty-nine years, died from a particularly virulent form of the disease, inflammatory breast carcinoma.

Hearing the Dread Diagnosis

Waiting in a doctor's office to learn the results of examinations for an ailment too painful or prominent to ignore, "you have cancer" is the diagnosis we all dread hearing. Most people tend to assume such a diagnosis is synonymous with a death sentence. And yet, thousands around the world do rid their bodies of cancer, especially those patients who venture beyond the confines of oncology treatment as it is now practiced in North America. You may be shocked when I reveal that some of the best natural and nontoxic therapies for healing cancer are not allowed to be administered in the United States or Canada because of misguided governmental regulations.

The book you are about to study contains educational information about cancer therapies practiced openly and legally in another technically advanced Western industrialized country: Germany. These practices may not be permitted in the United States or Canada. During the twentieth century, Germany's medical scientists developed anticancer treatments that are well known and respected. German oncologists are curing cancer patients without radical surgery, debilitating chemotherapy, or destructive radiation. Now that my father has written this book, cancer patients and their physicians on this side of the Atlantic can finally learn about successful cancer therapies formulated and practiced by oncologists in Germany.

Treatments German physicians are using enhance the human body's own inherent capacity to destroy malignant cells. These procedures are quite different from what the usual North American therapies provide. American and Canadian cancer treatments often are so toxic to the human body that they destroy many healthy cells along with the malignant cells, and result in terribly weakened immunity in the process. In contrast, many German cancer specialists have totally abandoned the usual, well-established, conventionally practiced procedures so as to avoid poisoning the patient. Rather, they have looked elsewhere and collected an oncological arsenal from around the world. Building on their past five decades of clinical usage, German doctors are now ready to proclaim their high success rates loudly and proudly and share what they've learned with the rest of the world.

The personal and professional relationship my father has had with numbers of innovative and successful German physicians over the past two decades has now enabled him to tell their story. Consequently, this book has been written for use by patients and medical professionals together.

Average American Doctors Seldom Know of German Therapies

Americans and Canadians may now fight off cancer without any need to surrender their bodies to blind faith in North American cookbook medicine. As a motivated, independent-minded patient, acting on information received on these pages, you can become empowered to choose safe, effective, natural, and nontoxic cancer therapies that have worked for people throughout Europe. As described, they are therapies that average American family physicians hardly ever offer. These doctors may not be aware of them.

You and your physician can now seek out anticancer alternatives, thanks to the German doctors who have shared their *Lebenswerk* (life work) with my father. Their successes can be your or your loved one's story too. A patient's fight against cancer need no longer involve having unquestioning confidence in the North American medical establishment, which has already lost the war against cancer; instead, it requires personal determination to find treatments applied overseas that have been beneficial for cancer patients among the dozen or more German-interpreting nations, such as Switzerland, Austria, Holland, and South Africa.

"Why," you might ask, "aren't the life-enhancing therapies being practiced by German doctors offered by physicians in the United States and Canada?" Dr. Walker lays out the reasons in his Introduction, which follows. Though it may seem odd, you can receive these German therapies in Tijuana, Mexico, a short drive from downtown San Diego, California. Although a Third World country, Mexico seems more open to investigating new techniques that overcome malignancies. Dr. Walker identifies and discusses a limited number of cancer treatments that are highly successful and recommended. By being informed about them, you will bring about a quicker arrival of existing therapeutic cancer breakthroughs on our side of the Atlantic.

Cancer therapy as practiced in North America relies primarily on attacking the human body with poisonous chemicals, burning it with radiation, or butchering its internal organs with a surgeon's knife. People everywhere are seeking refuge from this sort of vicious attack on their bodies. We intuitively believe there must be an alternative somewhere, if only we could find it. You will be able to do so now, with some of the therapies available in North America from the holistic physician members of the American College for Advancement in Medicine cited in Appendix B.

In the pages that follow, my father discusses seven highly effective alternative cancer therapies along with a bevy of worthwhile cancer marker tests. The treatments are derived from organic sources that enhance our bodies' own ability to fight cancerous cells. Based on interviews with German cancer specialists, searches of the worldwide cancer literature, visits to German cancer clinics and hospitals, and discussions with Americans and foreign nationals who have gone to Europe for treatment, along with treatment he has observed being rendered, Dr. Morton Walker knows that he is describing the future of oncology in North America, since these therapies already are showing effectiveness in Germany.

For most North Americans, it may be difficult to obtain some of the treatments not yet sanctioned by the American or Canadian medical establishments. The authorities that govern medicine on our continent will eventually recognize the excellent results achieved by German cancer specialists, but until then, the North American governments may present legal obstacles to obtaining the therapies about which you will learn. Additionally, unenlightened family physicians abetted by the American Cancer

Society and lobbyists representing the wealthiest of all indus-
tries, American pharmaceuticals, may try to avoid what German
oncologists are able to do. As potential cancer patients, however, none of us can afford to ignore the life-sustaining relief
mechanisms developed and perfected by German oncologists.
Indeed, by education and personal initiative, the lives we save
may be our own!

—Randall Scott Walker, C.P.A.

Introduction

My main admonition to any cancer patient from day one of our consultation is: "The best way to lose your battle with malignancy is to fall for the medical mainstream's aggressive cancer therapies before you've first undertaken the safer immune-supportive treatments of complementary and alternative medicine."

—My personal interview with Robert C. Atkins, M.D.,
New York City, January 12, 1998

Bringing people information about how they may prevent or fight off cancer is possibly the most important task of my life. I've seen too many friends and relatives, and my much loved wife, Joan, suffer terribly before finally succumbing to this disease. It has been my mission, regardless of cost or time, to uncover and report on anticancer therapies wherever they're to be found. My need is to reveal to everyone techniques of treatment that not only are effective and successful against cancer but also are the type that cause no torture for the hapless patient. Above all I have searched for remedies unabusive to or nonsuppressive of the human immune system, for this remarkably effective immunological organ brings about the ultimate healing.

I wish to offer cancer patients treatment choices, therapeutic options, and the resurgence of hope. Accordingly, my search has led me to discover that the innovative medical scientists and integrative health-care industry of Germany have developed or adopted effective ways of dealing with cancer. They go far beyond what is currently available in North America. Thus, my journalistic effort to bring you viable information about complementary and alternative natural and nontoxic cancer treatments finally has me feeling productive and rewarded. I have something positive to report.

Cancer patients are beginning to ward off their life-threatening conditions by becoming educated about the German cancer therapies discussed in the chapters to follow. Here I report on established medicinals, nutritionals, herbals, dietaries, and more that utilize effective healing methods for overcoming malignancies. The methods are gentle and don't consist of any carpet-bombing tactics for destroying cancer cells and healthy cells alike; rather, the effective procedures I've observed enhance an ill individual's immune system to eliminate offending cells that have refused to accept apoptosis (the body's normally programmed cellular death—cell suicide).

To illustrate such a procedure, for the first time ever this book provides information about Induced Remission Therapy (IRT). Having investigated IRT, German holisitic oncologists use this active cancer-reversing vaccine developed twenty years ago by a medical genius (who had become licensed as a medical doctor at only eighteen years of age). The inventor of IRT is an Australian physician, Samir "Dr. Sam" Chachoua, M.B., B.S. (see Chapter 10). Dr. Sam's IRT vaccine provides patients with far more permanent, less costly, and surer healing for greater numbers and types of cancers than do the currently touted Gleevec, Herceptin, Rituxan, Campath, C225, Iressa, and other pharmaceuticals offered by the international pharmaceutical industry as "breakthroughs." Rather, German medical specialists make ready use of the IRT vaccine to reverse the symptoms of cancer and acquired immunodeficiency syndrome (AIDS). I believe that only a few holistic physicians who use methods of complementary and alternative medicine and almost no conventionally practicing allopathic physicians in the United States ever have heard of Dr. Sam Chachoua's IRT.

Cancer Patients Worldwide Turn to CAM
for Treatment

An associate professor in the Department of Social Pharmacy at the Royal Danish School of Pharmacy, Laila Launso, M.Sc., D.Sc., has done extensive research on complementary and alternative medicine (CAM) techniques that are being used against malignancies. He finds that cancer patients worldwide have turned their attention to CAM for treatment. This new and startling development has occurred often without the treating oncologists even knowing that their patients are utilizing natural and nontoxic therapies (which Dr. Launso calls "unconventional cancer therapy," or UCT). The patients are employing UCT as an add-on to the doctors' usual conventional drug approaches for cancer.

According to Dr. Launso, UCT is widely used in Western countries. It is utilized by people from all socio-demographic groups and diagnosed with all types of cancer. Many of the people who turn to UCT want greater control of their treatment. Often, however, they are already in an advanced stage of their disease. On the whole, the patients trying UCT have reported a better general condition, tumors that have stopped growing or disappeared, and prevention of metastasis. According to Dr. Launso, "In some cases these outcomes have been documented by randomized clinical trials."[1]

The medical attitude toward UCT has varied among the different specialties and countries. "The dominating pattern is that knowledge about the usage and outcomes is very limited and more information is requested," says Dr. Launso.

Disenchantment of North American Cancer Patients

Medicine's allopathic entries in the anticancer sweepstakes—in particular chemotherapy and radiation therapy—really are crude disease-fighting weapons with limited effectiveness. North American cancer patients are known to fear them and mostly express disenchantment with the usual techniques of treatment. Because of the books and articles I write, people telephone me from around the world and from every state in the United States. They seek my advice about something new, something more in the battle for life against cancer. My heart goes out to them because I have been in their position. I went looking for something new, something more to save the life of my wife of forty-nine years.

The conventional weapons against cancer usually leave patients in a state of weakness, nauseated, bald, depressed, and otherwise uncomfortable. Practically none of these adverse effects occur when natural and nontoxic holistic therapies are integrated into a patient's treatment protocol.

One survey after another has made it abundantly clear that Americans and Canadians are disillusioned with the failing cancer therapies of mainstream drug-focused oncology. Almost everyone with medical insight acknowledges that the industrial/pharmaceutical/medical complex is incapable of or has no intention of providing any kind of curative procedure for cancer. My investigations have convinced me that this is true.

Still, we are fortunate in this wonderful country that our capitalistic system has allowed us a standard of living that is the envy of the rest of the world. Even with our good fortune, our system does contain some disadvantages such as the commercial companies that feel compelled to increase profits at the expense of the consumer. For a drug product to be developed, for instance, it must be patentable and profitable. If it is not, the public never is given access to it. That is the pathway for cancer too. Not finding appropriate and corrective cancer treatment tends to protect the income of the cancer establishment complex.

Until Now, the War on Cancer Has Been Lost

With our recent recognition that cancer is currently striking every second or third person in this country, we've had our eyes opened to the statements put out repeatedly by the American Cancer Society (ACS). I believe that the ACS has been less than truthful about the progress of cancer treatment solely for the purpose of raising funds. Since it seems to me that American medicine has been going in the wrong direction for over thirty years (since I began writing full-time), most of us realize that, until now, President Nixon's 1970s "War on Cancer" has been lost. And this loss probably happened even before it began.

The recommendations coming from the ACS do not merely include chemotherapy. The ACS also encourages patients to engage in radiation treatment. The ACS classifies radiation as a "proven" therapy when it appears to have *dis*proven itself repeatedly. I believe that radiation remains unsafe and is known to be a carcinogen that produces tissue burns, organ dysfunction, systemic sickness, and sometimes death. Its side effects are awful, something seldom told to medical consumers. Did you know, for example, that if your loved one has received radiation as treatment for breast cancer, her risk of undergoing coronary artery disease has increased fourfold?[2]

Where do we uncover the successful treatments against cancer and other life-threatening diseases? Surely they're not to be found at the neighborhood pharmacy or in our highly sophisticated hospitals that are filled with drug and radiation technology. And what remains for us—we, who are the loved ones left behind by those who have become the victims of cancer? I have agonized with the reality that no matter how much knowledge one holds or how many holistic physicians are prepared to help your beloved, you don't always win the battle with virulent cancer.

My Role as a Medical Journalist

I have been a medical journalist specializing in integrative methods of healing for overcoming all kinds of health problems for the past thirty-three years. My occupation has had me traveling to sixty-eight foreign nations among twenty-eight exotic cultures on six continents. From firsthand research, I have discovered that excellent natural and nontoxic therapies do exist. They lie awaiting our use everywhere except the United States and Canada. That's because the American pharmaceutical industry has its very own agenda. It has a powerful grip on the way medicine is practiced in North America—even in Mexico.

I have observed that most of American medical practice for treating cancer is *non*holistic and totally destructive. If, by chance, a therapeutic effect does result—well, that particular patient is just lucky to possess a strong immune system. Like some jar, crock, decanter, or amphora created through the skills of a potter, as described in Chapter 5 by German oncologist and Carnivora® developer Helmut Keller, M.D., the human immune system usually works when assisted by the correct remedies, which are nontoxic and natural. They are not drugs. Then the patient's immune defenses combined with therapy may be considered objects of beauty.

The Cancer Patient as an Object of Beauty

Keeping it as symmetrical as possible, the potter molds a clay pot into his or her desired shape. Any asymmetries are repaired so as to keep the pot balanced, and this is done by the potter working not only on any asymmetrical area but on the whole pot spinning on his wheel. The pot is in his or her hands going up and down for restoring balance. Treatment is rendered by that potter to the entire dynamic structure—the revolving pot on the potter's wheel—until it is perfect and the way it was envisioned.

In the hands of holistic oncologists—in this instance, those I have met in Germany—the cancer patient may be considered just such a pot, vessel, crock, amphora, or jar. When the patient's physician has fashioned a cancer protocol that is completely holistic (in that it almost exclusively includes natural and nontoxic remedies that do only good), treatment is rendered to the whole person. The therapy usually will vary in accordance with laboratory test results, clinical examinations, intuitive feelings, symptoms, and signs that may be ever changing, but the separate part or body system needing improvement is but one small portion of the complete individual. Permanent correction takes place only when the whole patient is corrected and balanced.

It seems to me that the image of a pot being thrown and turned into an object of beauty is a valid metaphor for the patient being restored to optimal health. Unlike conventionally practiced allopathic medicine, which follows cookbook procedures using toxic agents, holistic oncology utilizes safe, natural, and nonpoisonous treatments.

I have searched diligently for the appropriate cancer-healing remedies. Among all of the Western industrialized nations offering cancer patients nonsynthetic, nontoxic remedies such as the immunity-boosting tropical fruit extract noni (see Chapter 8) and the tumor-shrinking mushroom extract *Coriolus versicolor* (see Chapter 9), Germany stands out as open-minded and progressive.

Having traveled across the Atlantic at least two dozen times to interview German physicians about various holistic therapies, I have just drawn a mental parallel between the German holistic oncologist endeavoring to restore health to an endangered patient and the skillful potter throwing a pot to create a useful work of beauty.

Why We Need Natural and Nontoxic Cancer Therapies

Based on much preclinical testing and some human studies, not less than 135 natural and nontoxic cancer therapies are readily available for inhibiting cancer growths of all types. This book reports on 7 very important ones along with a series of hardly known cancer laboratory marker tests unrecognized in North America and restricted in their applications. Often the lab tests are employed by oncologists in German-speaking countries without governmental restriction. The remedies work by interfering with metabolic mechanisms central to cancer progression. And the benefits of those 135 medical devices, herbs, enzymes, hormones, nutrients, nutriceuticals, and other agents are likely to be more therapeutic when used in large combinations for their synergistic interactions.

North Americans are steadily becoming enlightened about the integrated cancer therapies accessible to them.[3,4] With the cooperation of trained health professionals, the public wants the ability to choose its own form of treatment. My intention is to educate people to the fact that excellent anticancer therapies do exist, albeit not yet in the United States and Canada. They may be applied for reducing the burdens that cancer inflicts on ourselves and the people whom we love. My anticipation is that in some small measure I have achieved this intent. In such a manner patients who have malignancies may realize that choices of treatment do present themselves.

With the medical journalistic work I have invested in this book and the reportage of other investigators who write, the education of those people with life-threatening disease has only just begun. The therapies reported on here are Polyerga® in Chapters 1 and 2; Carnivora® in Chapters 3, 4, and 5; galvanotherapy in Chapter 6; hyperthermia in Chapter 7; noni in Chapter 8; *Coriolus versicolor* in Chapter 9; and Induced Remission Therapy in Chapter 10. There are many other treatments that definitely need exposure too. They are not included in this modest effort. Among the additional German cancer therapies that I or another medical journalist will eventually get to discuss in forthcoming books are the following:

Antineoplaston therapy	Chaparral
Hydrazine sulfate	Dr. Moerman's anticancer diet
Livingston therapy	DMSO/hematoxylon therapy
Hoxsey therapy	Mind/body therapies
Pau d'arco	Nutritional therapy
Wheatgrass therapy	Revici therapy
Chelation therapy	Essiac
Homeopathy	Mistletoe (Iscador®)
Chinese medicine	Macrobiotics
Gaston Naessen's 714-X	Oxygen therapies
Lawrence Burton's immuno-	Live-cell therapy
augmentative therapy	Ayurveda
Dr. Issel's whole-body therapy	Enderlein therapy
Gerson therapy	

In the above listing, mistletoe (iscador®) therapy stands out because of a major thirty-year-long study on over 35,000 residents of Heidelberg, Germany, 5,000 of whom had cancer. "Mistletoe is the most commonly used cancer drug in Germany today," says David Riley, M.D., editor in chief of *Alternative Therapies in Health and Medicine*, publisher of the study. This publication has been a leading peer-reviewed American journal on complementary and alternative medicine. The study, *"Viscum Album* in Cancer Treatment: A Systematic Epidemiology Investigation," showed that mistletoe extract greatly improves survival rate for a wide variety of cancers. Users lived 40 percent longer compared with those who did not ingest the plant. The researchers matched more than 300 pairs of participants who were the victims of similar types and stages of disease. One group took mistletoe extract in addition to conventional treatment. After comparing the length of patient survival, the study concluded that those who added mistletoe extract to their treatment lived a two-fifths longer period than those who did not.[5]

The Author's Goal for This Book

I want you to know of my goal as the author of this health book. It follows an overriding theme. My aim is to inform medical consumers everywhere about the 7 remedies described in the following chapters. Also I want to leave you with an awareness that lots of other treatment methods exist. There are a great number of other complementary and alternative methods of healing cancer as well, and often they are superior to the conventional oncological therapies commonly offered in North America. Find them, use them, and save your life.

PART ONE

Polyerga®

This section has been written in consultation with
Dr. Martin Klingmueller, Rer. Ter. Nat., and
Dr. Jurgen Kuhlmey, B.Ecc., M.Sc., Ph.D.

1

Properties of Polyerga®

When in 1967, Irmgard M., a bank teller living in Bremen, Germany, was forty-eight years old, her steadily increasing voice roughness and breathing difficulties finally became intolerable. Frau M. acknowledged that the two packs of cigarettes she had been smoking daily for twenty years were a probable cause, but she remained unprepared for the histologically confirmed laryngeal cancer that became her diagnosis. Confined to a single site on the glottis, her tumor was judged by the oncologists conducting her X-ray examination, blood tests, manual palpation, and biopsy to be a Stage I (T1) squamous cell carcinoma.

In the biopsy procedure that she underwent, a piece of the tumor was surgically removed and examined under the microscope. In that way the cancer's true diagnosis and staging could be identified. By means of standard oncological treatment, the five-year survival for a person with this malignant condition has been declared by prior cancer statistics as approximately 75 percent. On average, therefore, Irmgard M. was given three chances out of four of living five years more.

To assure this chance for Frau M., the attending oncologist prescribed surgery and follow-up chemotherapy. During July of that same year she did undergo cordectomy of the right vocal cord, and the surgeon observed no metastases to surrounding tissues. But after follow-up cytotoxic therapies with the two anticancer chemicals cisplatin and 5-fluorouracil (5-FU), various adverse side effects set in that kept her uncomfortable for twelve months.

During that first year of follow-up, the patient returned to work and did continue uneventfully for five years thereafter without recurrence. Because of that five-year timing, Frau M.'s doctors advised that a "cure" had been achieved, and she was given a clean bill of health. Unfortunately, the patient's advisers were wrong!

Although Irmgard M. had stopped smoking upon being diagnosed and did not resume the practice, by May 1973 a worsening hoarseness and breathing problem caused her to undergo another biopsy of the voice box. A lentil-size tumor was present; her cancer had returned. The biopsy report from Bremen pathologist Myer Loman, M.D., stated: "Microscopically observed is excised tumor tissue containing undifferentiated carcinoma cells with significant polymorphic nuclei all of which is attached to connective tissue."

The presence of undifferentiated carcinoma cells indicates that Frau M. possessed malignant cellular tissue that did not particularly look like the normal tissue it came from. Rather the tissue cells appeared primitive or immature. Such undifferentiated or poorly differentiated tumor material tends to be more aggressive in its behavior. The primitive cells grow faster, spread earlier, and have a worse prognosis than well-differentiated tumors.[1]

Even being made aware of this dangerous cellular characteristic, Frau M. refused the surgeon-professor's request for a return visit to the hospital to go through the removal of her entire larynx. Such an excision would have eliminated her ability to speak altogether, and she wanted nothing to do with any kind of permanent silence.

When I interviewed her at home in Bremen in April 2001,

Irmgard M. told me, "The surgeon attempted to persuade me to have the operation. He warned me that steady enlargement of the tumor mass in my throat would block breathing and interfere with my capacity to inhale air. Thus, he said, I must eventually die from asphyxiation or heart attack. Even so, I still refused the operation," Frau M. declared. "I did not want to live the rest of my life without the ability to speak.

"Upon explaining to my family doctor about this death sentence that the surgeon pronounced on me, my doctor told me of possible treatment by another doctor, the renowned oncology researcher Professor Walter Kuhlmey, M.D., Ph.D. He was also located in Bremen. So I phoned and made an appointment for a medical consultation the next morning," advises Frau M. "Dr. Kuhlmey took my medical history, examined me, and then stated: 'If you do what I direct you to do, I will get you through this malignancy.'

"So I followed his instructions faithfully. From Dr. Walter Kuhlmey I received an injection of Polyerga® liquid every morning and swallowed Polyerga Plus™ tablets several times each day throughout the week. Continuing such treatment for six weeks, I felt much better and spoke with less roughness in my voice. I was happy with my progress and decided to show my family doctor how I was coming along," Frau M. says. "When he looked down my throat with his lighted instrument he was amazed to see that the redness was gone and the tumor had shrunk. Later I learned that my doctor had been so impressed by what he saw that he was prescribing the same kind of Polyerga Plus™ tablets for his other patients who were suffering with various forms of cancer.

"Next I traveled to Hamburg, where still another cancer surgeon examined my throat while I was under the effects of narcosis. During our consultation later, this surgeon offered to cut a small window through my larynx so that I could breathe as the small tumor that was left grew larger. The surgeon had no idea about how Polyerga® worked and that it was helping me. Therefore, I refused the window-cutting procedure. I was pleased with how Polyerga® had been shrinking the tumor and preferred to stay with this pig spleen extract as my only form of required treatment," states Frau M. "Polyerga® is the single form of medicine that I've taken as a preventive measure against cancer for the past thirty years. It has been successful for me all of this time, and I see no reason to deviate from such a course of action."

No surgery, chemotherapy, or radiation therapy has ever been required by this patient from the moment she began taking regular injections and nutritional supplements with the porcine spleen extract. Frau Irmgard M.'s laryngeal carcinoma did not worsen thereafter. With the expectation of living into her nineties, she currently undergoes regular semiannual physical and laboratory examinations.

The patient's elevated cancer markers had fallen to normal at the beginning of porcine spleen treatment and have remained that way, indicating that her immune system has stabilized and beneficial biological response modification is settled in. Until today, 1 ml of subcutaneous Polyerga® per week plus 100 mg of oral Polyerga® in tablet or capsule form have been continued. She gives the treatment to herself. Her hoarseness is gone, breathing is easy, and she enjoys a high quality of life in all respects. While I interviewed Frau Irmgard M. for writing this book chapter, she served me tea, homemade cookies, and a delicious whole-grain brown bread spread with strawberry jam that she also had made. She sent me home to Stamford, Connecticut, with a jar of the jam.

Polyerga® Promotes Remission of Stomach Cancer

During the fall of 1990, a second oncology patient, Franz L., who was then eighty-one years old and retired as a high school principal in the Hanover, Germany, public school system, was experiencing gradually worsening pain in the low back, chest, and upper abdomen. Over time, Herr L. also developed symptoms similar to hiatal hernia or peptic ulcer, namely nausea, heartburn, and indigestion aggravated to the point of severe discomfort by eating almost any food. He self-treated his discomforts with antacids, which offered some temporary relief but not much. Simultaneously black stools appeared any time he defecated. After a short time, he went through a period of appetite loss, feelings of fullness after consuming even a small meal, and a noticeable weight loss.

When, in early 1991, his weight had fallen by more than 10 percent, Herr L. consulted a Hanover gastroenterologist, who ordered laboratory tests, performed an X-ray study, and conducted a clinical examination on him. The patient showed blood in his stools, anemia from gastrointestinal bleeding, a high level of carcinoembryonic antigen (CEA), an elevated amount of serum ferritin, and achlorhydria. Roentgenological examination of the upper gastrointestinal tract uncovered a large ulcerlike lesion. On palpation, he exhibited enlarged lymph nodes above the left collarbone (supraclavicular node), nodal masses around the rectum, an oversized liver (hepatomegaly), and increased abdominal fluid (ascites). A follow-up gastroscopic examination resulted in a diagnosis of carcinoma of the stomach.

One month later Franz L. underwent an exploratory gastric surgery in which the stomach surgeons observed a walnut-sized neoplasm. They took specimens for biopsy, and the subsequent diagnosed malignancy was judged inoperable. No liver metastases could be found. Chemotherapy for the stomach cancer was recommended, but Herr L. preferred a type of treatment that encompasses complementary and alternative medicine (CAM). Therefore he sought the services of a holistic physician who utilized oncological nondrug CAM methods—techniques of healing that are noninvasive, nontoxic, natural, immune stimulating, and nonharmful in any way.

From day one of consultation with his holistic physician, Franz

L. received twice-daily administration (morning and evening) of effective subcutaneous (SC) injections of 1 ml of Polyerga®. When, after four weeks, he was released from the CAM oncologist's care with normal cancer marker tests, he continued Polyerga® treatment on his own at home. Herr L. gave himself a 1-ml subcutaneous injection into the skin of his abdominal area every other day for twenty days; then for one year he injected 1 ml of the porcine spleen extract into his own buttock twice per week. Afterward dosage reduction was made to a single ml of the SC injection per week for another year.

Also as part of his usual daily nutritional supplementation, Herr L. swallowed one Polyerga® tablet (Polyerga Plus™) three times a day with meals. Each tablet offered him a dosage of 100 mg of porcine spleen oligopeptides. If he had been inclined to utilize Polyerga® capsules instead, Herr L. would have been receiving 100 mcg of porcine spleen glycopeptides, recommended to be taken as a single capsule once every other day with meals. The product's German manufacturer, HorFerVit Pharma GmbH of Oldenburg, Germany, makes it in two oral forms, capsules and tablets.

No chemotherapy had ever been administered to Franz L. during the eight years he was victimized by the stomach malignancy. He eventually did die in 1998 at age eighty-nine but not from gastric cancer. That malignant condition he had survived without difficulty. Rather, Franz L. succumbed to complications associated with the trauma of falling from horseback while out riding with his great-grandchildren.

Defining the Peptides in Porcine Spleen Polyerga®

What are the ingredients present in Polyerga® that restored health to elderly Franz L., and to Frau Irmgard M., who is now eighty-one years old but who arrived on the cancer scene before him? The vital substances are peptide growth factors, molecular chains of amino acids, which are constituents of every animal organ. They are composed of the tiniest of protein molecules, which biochemists and physiologists call *peptides*. Certain protein growth factors present in porcine (pork) spleen possess beneficial characteristics for the treatment of cancer and other degenerative diseases in animals other than pigs and in human beings too.

The dalton, a measurement of molecular weight, has been assigned the symbol of D or Da (also called an *atomic mass unit*). A dalton is equivalent to 1.657×10^{-24} gm. Porcine spleen peptides, the therapeutic components of Polyerga®, are of a low molecular weight (1,500 Da) and, on hydrolysis, yield up to a maximum of one hundred sequential peptide molecules. Although scientists have so far been unable to determine their sequence, these one hundred pig spleen peptides are composed of ten amino acids in a chain, which defines them as a *polypeptide*.

Peptide growth factors in nearly all animal organs form by loss of water from the NH_2 and COOH molecular groups of adjacent amino acids and are additionally referred to by biochemists as di-, tri-, tetra-, etc. peptides, depending on the number of amino acids in the molecule. Thus peptides come together as polypeptides, larger in size than a peptide, but smaller than a protein. They form by the partial breakdown of proteins or by connecting amino acids into chains to make up the constituent parts of proteins.

According to which of the various scientific disciplines are being queried, different names exist for peptide growth factors. Historically, for instance, cell biologists have called members of their identified growth factor–type set of molecules *growth factors;* immunologists have named their growth factor types *interleukins, lymphokines,* or *cytokines;* while hematologists have used the growth factor-type descriptive term *colony-stimulating factors* (CSF). However, the present generally delineating nomenclature for peptides is *growth factors,* and the term has been and is now widely used throughout the world's scientific literature.

The *growth factor* term is applied consistently among most scientific and medical disciplines because in nearly every case it reflects the context of the original discovery or isolation of any peptide. Since essentially all of these many molecules are multi-functional, it's not easy to conceive of unique new names for them that would be entirely satisfactory; almost all of them are "panregulins," that is, they react as universal regulators of the particular organ from which they derive.[2]

In this case, Polyerga® is just such a panregulin purified and processed in a patented unique manner by HorFerVit Pharma GmbH of Oldenburg, Germany, from the spleen of the pig. The product has shown itself to be a regulator or stabilizer of the immune system. For the animal and human body, panregulins as peptide growth factors are physiological symbols for the transfer of signals or a kind of language of biological regulation/stabilization.[3]

Peptides often promote cell growth, but they also can inhibit it; moreover, they regulate or stabilize many critical cellular functions, such as in the control of cell differentiation and other processes which have little to do with growth itself. All peptide growth factors act in sets. To understand their actions, one must always consider the biological context in which they act.

Peptide growth factors provide an essential means for each cell to communicate with its immediate environment. They ensure that there is proper local homeostatic balance between the numerous cells that compose a tissue or organ. Since a cell must adjust its behavior to changes in its environment, the cell needs mechanisms to provide this adaptation. The tissue cells either singularly or collectively, therefore, use sets of peptide growth factors as signaling molecules to communicate with each other and to alter their own behavior to respond appropriately to their biological context. Such signaling within the confines of an individual's immune system encourages homeostatic stabilization.

The peptide growth factors of pig spleen that make up Polyerga® act by binding to functional receptors which transduce their signals, and the peptides themselves may be viewed as bifunctional molecules. Three main responses or actions that pig spleen peptide growth factors accomplish are:

1. They possess an afferent function in that there is the conveying of information to cellular receptors, providing them with information from outside the animal or human organism's cell, tissue, or organ.

2. They have an efferent function in that there is the inception of any latent biochemical activity of the receptor.

3. They offer up physiological symbols of communication within the organ systems of nearly all animal and human organisms.

These peptides possess the unique action of serving as a significant means to convey information from one cell to another or from one organ to the next, including the brain and central nervous system, and their action in this regard is contextual, meaning that they weave together the person's organ actions even in the presence of a degenerative disease such as cancer.

Pig Spleen Peptides Improve the Quality of Life for Cancer Patients

Manufactured under the Polyerga® brand name, peptides of low molecular weight taken from the pig (porcine) spleen improve immune system reactivity and the quality of life for patients suffering from malignancies. This circumstance was especially apparent in 158 breast cancer patients who were losing weight and failing in health after treatment with standard oncological therapies. The patients definitely had shown a decreased performance status and suppressed immunological parameters. But administering Polyerga® to them stabilized the patients' immune systems so well that their appetites improved to the point that all of them regained lost weight, restored their immunoreactivity, and caused them to experience a measurable increase in the release of their impaired mitogen-induced gamma-interferon (g-IFN) by peripheral blood lymphocytes.[4]

Allow me to explain the above statement in clearer detail: Immune system stabilization by use of Polyerga® was proven by three oncologists at Klinik Sonnenblick located in Marburg, Germany, in 1995. Then, 158 breast cancer patients in an open controlled trial were divided by the three physicians into two groups. The women in Group A were administered 1 ml of the described porcine spleen low-molecular-weight glycopeptide extract by SC injection three times per week without any other anticancer or immune medication. In comparison, another set of breast cancer patients in Group B were administered SC injections of vitamins and minerals. Before this study began for both groups, the immunoreactivity of the patients had been suppressed, and all of them were recorded as at least 20 percent underweight. Various parameters were measured for these two groups, but the patients treated with Polyerga® improved far in excess of the controls.

In the Polyerga®-treated Group A, the patients' diagnostic assays revealed a great deal. Their percentage of blood lymphocytes, Merieux skin tests, Karnofsky performance status, and sense of well-being increased significantly more as compared to the control Group B.[5]

Years back, working together with his now deceased physician/chemist father, Walter Kuhlmey, M.D., Ph.D., and his biochemist brother, Jurgen Kuhlmey, B.Ecc., M.Sc., Ph.D. (who actively manages their HorFerVit Pharma GmbH company), Kristian Kuhlmey, M.D., had perfected the therapeusis of Polyerga® from porcine spleen which yields the above-described oligopeptides GP-1. As mentioned, these peptides are both immune stabilizers and biologic response modifiers.

In laboratory investigations, the Polyerga® peptides have been proven to increase the survival rate of mice that had been infected with the influenza A virus[6] as well as for relieving the suffering of humans who are infected by chronic hepatitis B.[7]

Applied for the improvement of the quality of life in head and neck cancer patients while they were receiving chemotherapy with cytotoxin 5-FU and cisplatin derivations, Polyerga® became good supportive treatment. Proof of this support manifested itself in a randomized, placebo-controlled, double-blind clinical study conducted on forty participating patients. Twenty of the patients received 1-ml SC injections of Polyerga® and another twenty received SC injections merely containing placebo. During their cytotoxic treatments, lymphocyte counts of the group of Polyerga®-treated patients stabilized significantly. In comparing the two groups, the investigators confirmed that their placebo-treated patients did not stabilize at all.[8]

Moreover, the chemically pretreated patients experienced a lessening of fatigue and greater elevation of their energy levels when given SC injections of pig spleen peptides.

Approved by the Food and Drug Administration of Germany (but not the USFDA as yet), Polyerga® is backed by additional quantities of randomized, controlled, double-blind clinical studies on patients and by numbers of laboratory experiments on animals (please see the international studies described below).

Clinical Studies of Polyerga® Conducted in Two Balkan Countries

In German clinical practice at the former oncology clinic and hospital, Bad Wiessee's Klinik Winnerhof (now closed), the product had been employed by Dr. Kristian Kuhlmey (now deceased) to stabilize cancer patients' immune systems, raise their survival ability, enhance the quality of life, and improve their compliance with radiation therapy and/or chemotherapy when such a modality is mandatory.

Definitely observed by clinical oncologists is that the Polyerga® peptides:

- act as suppressors of tumor cell growth
- stimulate lymphocyte proliferation
- excite lymphocyte response
- elevate immune status for patients pretreated with chemotherapy
- reduce melanoma and lung cancer metastases

At the Department of Experimental Biology and Medicine of the Rudjer Boskovic Institute in Zagreb, Croatia, Polyerga® was applied in laboratory and clinical investigations. It decreased the number of experimental lung metastases in mice, and the substance was also used during supportive treatment of tumorous patients. In their conclusion, the investigators wrote: "With Polyerga®, a pronounced stimulation of the host's immune reactivity on the one hand and a significant tumor mass reduction on the other were determined repeatedly."[9]

Next, the same group of Croatian experimenters studied the influence of chemotherapy with cyclophosphamide cytotoxic agent and/or spleen peptides on the incidence of experimental lung metastases of breast cancer in mice. They found that the oral application of Polyerga® was significantly more effective in reducing the number of lung metastases than the application of chemotherapy alone. The researchers concluded: "Polyerga® preparation is active against tumor metastases, particularly if combined with the standard chemotherapy."[10]

At that same Rudjer Boskovic Institute, another study, this one supported by the Croatian Ministry of Science and Technology, was conducted to learn if mice bearing artificial lung metastases of mammary carcinoma responded positively to Polyerga®. They did! When the porcine spleen oligopeptides were combined with a dose of chemotherapy (Endoxan 50 mg/kg single intraperitoneal dose), the average metastatic development was four times lower than in the control mice treated by chemotherapy alone. Compared to all of the control animals, which died from their cancers within forty-two days when they were treated only with chemotherapy, just half of the chemo/ Polyerga®-treated mice died by the end of forty-two days. "Thus, these results give an experimental support for the use of the porcine spleen peptides in biotherapy (or combined therapy) of cancer," stated the Croatian medical researchers.[11]

In another Balkan country, two medical research facilities, the Clinic of Gastroenterology, Department of Internal Diseases, Medical University at the Sofia University Hospital "Saint Iv. Rilskii" and the National Institute for Infectious and Parasitic Diseases, Virological Laboratory of Sofia, both in Bulgaria, cooperated in a study of Polyerga®. This Bulgarian research was focused on the effects of low-molecular-weight glycoproteins from pig spleen in the treatment of ten patients with biopsy-proven chronic hepatitis B virus (HBV) showing ongoing infection replication. Intramuscular injections of Polyerga® were administered to the infected people three times per week. Also, three tablets of the pork peptides were dispensed daily for twenty-four weeks to these same patients. The effect on viral replication was evaluated by measuring HBV-DNA and HbeAg in serum for alanine aminotransferase (ALT).

As a result of this treatment, in three out of the ten virally infected patients HBV-DNA became undetectable and the pathological ALT decreased. The Bulgarian investigators advised, "The effect of increasing the cytolysis shows that the Polyerga® drug is active, probably by increasing the lymphokine secretion and the generation of cytotoxic T-cells. The absence of side effects plus its ability to reduce viral replication and lower ALT activity even in patients with liver cirrhosis warrants further studies of Polyerga® as an [adjunctive] 'second drug' or as a drug of choice [for Hepatitis B]."[12]

The Pork Peptide Product Studied in Canada

At the Montreal General Hospital in Montreal, Quebec, Canada, oncologists utilized Polyerga® for twenty-five patients who were close to death from advanced cancer. These were unfortunate people for whom no other therapeutic agent had proven effective. Use of the pork peptide substance in a Phase I–II study was cleared by the Canadian Health Protection Branch (Canada's FDA) and the hospital's Institutional Review Board.

The Polyerga® peptides were administered to these twenty-five patients by tablet three times a day and SC injection three times per week. No adverse side effects were experienced, but no significant hematological or biochemical changes were detected, except that one of the patients experienced the stabilization of his disease.

For these cancer patients who were exceedingly close to death, the median length of survival from the start of their oncologists giving Polyerga® turned out to be 102 days. The longest survivor lived for seventy-seven weeks (529 days). At the conclusion of their published paper, the doctors reported, "Polyerga® is safe but more studies are needed to determine its anticancer effects."[13]

Spanish Oncologists Use Polyerga® as a Biologic Response Modifier

In Madrid, Spain, at the Centro de Investigaciones Biologicas, C.S.I.C., eight oncology researchers had used Polyerga® for cancer patients as a biologic response modifier (BMR). Reporting in *Research and Experimental Medicine*, the investigators sought to prove that treatment with porcine spleen peptides can increase the number of plaque-forming cells and rosette-forming cells, as well as improve the reduced mitogen-induced gamma-IFN (g-IFN) release in peripheral blood cells from cancer patients.

The researchers acknowledge that "treatment with Polyerga® can increase appetite, body weight, performance status, and subjective well-being in cancer patients. An improvement of immunoreactivity of cancer patients during Polyerga® treatment also occurs." Hence, in the hands of the Spanish oncologists, Polyerga® delivered a biologic response modifying effect for their patients tantamount to immune stabilization.

Using the same sort of pig spleen peptides, these particular Spanish oncologists conducted in vivo laboratory experiments. They undertook to prove the reported BRM-like human clinical responses of Polyerga® in laboratory mice, and they succeeded.[14]

The Attributes of Biologic Response Modifiers

To provide functional immunological support for patients with cancerous tumors, numerous *biologic response modifiers* (BRMs) have been utilized by progressive oncology therapists who practice complementary and alternative medicine. BRMs and CAM are synergistic for each other with every cancer patient. Moreover, the therapist attending to each cancer patient discovers that there ultimately are healing benefits for the patient by such synergism. BRMs are an optimal form of biological therapy.

Based on a proven concept that the human immune system is designed to eliminate and destroy any foreign substances such as bacteria and viruses inside the body, biological therapy has come to fruition during the past decade. While difficulties may remain from the patient's physiology not recognizing malignant cells as foreign body substances, such problems are steadily being overcome as a result of medical research. Great strides in this direction have been made by applying highly purified proteins which we know are *peptides*. They activate the immune system so it works more effectively. Interferon and interleukin-2 have been the best known of these protein peptides, but there are dozens of other similar biological immune system enhancement agents as well. Nearly all biologic response modifiers exhibit four main attributes. The BRMs:[15]

1. directly trigger or stimulate an involved person's immune system

2. offer tumor management by indirectly shrinking or destroying malignant growth

3. advantageously modulate the activities of hormones, enzymes, and other biological components

4. contribute to permanent malignancy remission

American oncologist Douglas Brodie, M.D., of Reno, Nevada, utilizes vast numbers of BRMs for bolstering the body's natural immune defenses against cancer. These include nutrients and other food factors, as well as hormones and special immune-modulating substances. (For a list of these substances, see "Biological Immune System Enhancement Agents" below and on pages 29–30.) "My main objective over the past two decades has been to find those natural substances that most effectively enhance the immune system in its battle against cancer," says Dr. Brodie. "When these substances are part of a comprehensive cancer treatment plan, which includes strong physical and psychological support, the chances of beating cancer are markedly improved."[16]

Biological Immune System Enhancement Agents

Tumor-cell-modulating immunotherapy employs biological agents such as the interferons.[17] All types of immunotherapy depend on the patient's immune cells recognizing malignant cells. The only way they can do this is by spotting certain antigens on the surface of cancer cells, which is a somewhat difficult task. A standard term used in oncology, *cell modulation,* means that tumor-associated antigens become highlighted so as to give the patient's immune system cells a cleaner target to aim for.

Over the past decade, diverse biological agents and many approaches to biological therapy have been investigated by oncology scientists. Typical of more than five dozen natural, refined, or otherwise manufactured immune system enhancement agents derived from both plant and animal sources and in use today are the following:

Porcine spleen peptides/
    Polyerga®
Antineoplastons
Bovine thymus extract/NatCell™
Porcine and bovine liver extract
Bovine tracheal cartilage
Phytochemicals
Crude bacteria
Cytokines other than those
    cited here
Shark cartilage
Interleukins
Interferons
Colony-stimulating factors
Glandular and organ extracts
Harvested T-lymphocytes
Tumor necrosis factors
Gene therapy
Alkylglycerols/shark liver oil
Antiangiogenesis factors
Monoclonal antibodies
Human mother's breast milk
Dimethyl sulfoxide (DMSO)
Camphor and organic salts/714X®
Homeopathic-potentized
    nucleic acids

Venus' flytrap extract/
    Carnivora®
Hansi homeopathic activator
Chlorella
Sea vegetables
Green concentrates
Aloe vera
Amygdalin/laetrile
Astragalus
Cat's claw/uña de gato
Echinacea
Essiac
Flavonoids
Garlic
Gingko biloba
Ginseng/*Panax*
Oligomeric proanthocyanidin/
    OPC®
Grape seed extract/Pycnogenol®
Green tea/catechins
Haelan® 951
Hoxsey herbs
Mistletoe/Iscador®
Larch arabinogalactan/
    Larix®, ARA-6®
Maitake mushroom/*Grifola*

Sodium butyrate

Hydrazine sulfate

Glutathione/Immunocal®

Staphage lysate

Dr. Pekar's autologous vaccine

Coley's toxins

Immuno-augmentative therapy

TVZ-7 lymphocyte treatment

Anti-mycoplasma auto-vaccine

Enderlein/pleomorphic remedies

Melatonin

Autologous vaccine

Pau d'arco/lapacho

Modified citrus pectin

Silymarin/milk thistle

Turmeric

Ukrain

Urea

Bacillus Calmette-Guerin
   vaccine

T/Tn antigen breast cancer
   vaccine

Immunoplacental therapy

Oxygen therapies

BRM Studies of Polyerga® Conducted in Germany

At the Medizinische Klinik der Ruhr-Universitaet of Bochum in Germany and the St. Josef Hospital in Bochum, three different biologic response modifiers, thymopentin (TP5), factor AF2, and Polyerga®, were tested and compared in twenty-three healthy humans and twenty-three cancer patients. Each of the BRMs significantly released interferon-g (g-IFN), but Polyerga® influenced early T-cell and B-cell differentiation for the cancer patients. There was significant restoration of their impaired g-IFN production, which is important because g-IFN is a key cytokine in T-cell macrophage communication. Reduction of g-IFN concentration as a response to the stimulatory signal causes a profound inhibition of subsequent immune reactions.[18]

At the LPT Laboratory of Pharmacology and Toxicology in Hamburg, Germany, a whole range of toxicological studies were conducted on Polyerga® solution prepared for injection. The product's LD_{50} in rats (the toxic dosage reached when half the laboratory animals die) was determined as 3.76 b.w. milliliters per kilogram (ml/kg) of body weight intravenously. There was no toxicity up to a dose level of 2 ml/kg b.w./day during the thirteen-week treatment period. The several embryotoxicity studies showed no teratogenic properties and no mutagenic potential. The maximum therapeutic dose is at least fifty times the standard dose of three times 1 ml per week. Polyerga® therefore provides a wide margin of safety at the therapeutic dose levels.[19]

Conducted at two German tumor centers, one in Munich and the other in Oldenburg, recent clinical trials of Polyerga® for the treatment of metastasized colon cancer in forty patients indicates that their survival was significant. That's because this was a randomized, placebo-controlled, double-blind study in which one group of twenty patients received Polyerga® and the other group of twenty received placebo.

In 1977, at the Krankenhaus Deisterhort (Deisterhort Hospital) in Bad Munder, Germany, two groups of twenty patients, each having stomach cancer, participated in a prospective, randomized, placebo-controlled, double-blind study of Polyerga® injections. The patients in Group A received the Polyerga® treatment, and the Group B patients were the controls who received only a liver extract. Then the results of Group A and Group B were matched which revealed that the porcine spleen peptides allowed patients to survive considerably longer. In fact, among the treated patients 44 percent lived for at least five years compared to only 11 percent of the control patients.

The authors of this investigation wrote, "The results of the prospective randomized study justify the recommendation of Polyerga® treatment of carcinoma of the stomach, which should start immediately after the diagnosis."[20]

By itself, Polyerga® is unable to induce lymphocyte proliferation; rather, it needs a cofactor called concanavalin A (ConA), a phytochemical derived from the jack bean plant or *Canavalia ensiformis*. ConA is known to possess mitogenic activity and stimulates lymphocyte proliferation on its own. In an experiment carried out by one of this book's consultants, Dr. Martin Klingmueller, production manager of HorFerVit Pharma GmbH, human lymphocytes were stimulated at a low level by ConA and Polyerga® in combination, but such stimulation was solely dependent on the concentration of Polyerga® peptides. There was strictly a dose-effect relationship. This means that Polyerga® works only in combination with other factors and no overstimulation of the immune system can be induced. Such a significant circumstance is vital in immune therapy.[21]

Resources

Polyerga® is distributed throughout North America under a licensure agreement that comes from the product's German manufacturer, HorFerVit Pharma GmbH, located at Heinrich-Brockmann Strasse (Street) 81 or Post Office Box (Postfach) 2329; D-26131 Oldenburg, Germany; telephone 011(49)441-350 330 or 011(49)441-503036; fax 011(49)441-506610 or 011(49)441-350 3333; e-mail horfervit-pharma@t-online.de; website http://www.horfervit.de.

The SC, IM, and IV porcine spleenic injectables of Polyerga® are not approved for North American distribution by either the Canadian Health Protection Branch or the U.S. Food and Drug Administration. The exclusive licensee granted distribution rights by HorFerVit Pharma GmbH in the United States for Polyerga Plus™ tablets and capsules is Southeastern Health Products, Inc., 1 Johnston Street, Suite 15, Corporate Row, Savannah, Georgia 31405; telephone (800) 382-2438; fax (912) 352-2399; e-mail southeasternhp@aol.com; no website is available at this time.

The exclusive United States distributor of Polyerga® is European Lifestyle Products, LLC, P.O. Box 1345, Gibsonia, Pennsylvania 15044; telephone (724) 934-3068; fax (724) 934-9181; e-mail elp@zoominternet.net; website http://www.european lifestyleproducts.com.

2

Anticancer Effects of Polyerga®

By the mid-1930s, Professor Walter Kuhlmey, M.D., Ph.D., was already well established as an oncological researcher and clinician in the medical facilities of the most famous German surgeon of his day, Professor Ferdinand Sauerbruch, M.D. Dr. Sauerbruch, known as "the master surgeon" (which was also the title of his self-published autobiography), had invented the pressure chamber, an apparatus that saved countless lives in the field of chest surgery. As apprentices, Dr. Sauerbruch took in only the most brilliant medical scholars to work in his vast clinic and hospital.

After achieving all that he had wanted as an oncology clinician studying under "this master surgeon," Dr. Walter Kuhlmey turned his attention to drug manufacturing in his own factory in Berlin. He specialized in producing insulin for the medical needs of German diabetics. After World War II had begun, Dr. Kuhlmey was ordered by the Nazi government to move his pharmaceutical plant to Oldenburg, Germany, where multiple slaughterhouses were located. The slaughterhouses could furnish him with domestic animal organs from which he could extract insulin. When his plant was bombed and burned to the ground in 1944, he was forced to close down and await the war's termination. He conducted a clinical cancer practice during this waiting period.

Then, he again built a pharmaceutical enterprise, specializing in insulin production. But sources of insulin from pancreas tissues were difficult to come by, because during the postwar period there was a shortage of domestic animals, especially pigs. Consequently, the senior Dr. Kuhlmey attempted to produce insulin from other animal organs, specifically from the spleen of calves (bovine) and pigs (porcine). Pig spleen peptides evolved most readily as a semi-substitute source of insulin which caused no adverse reactions when Dr. Kuhlmey experimented with them on his own body. Instead, the pig spleen peptides offered pain relief, a sense of well-being, more energy, and less fatigue. He named his new product Polyerga® (from the Latin, *poly* meaning "multiple" and *erga* referring to "power" or "potent").

One day in 1951, Julia M., a sixty-year-old patient with far advanced pancreatic cancer, was being treated by the Oldenburg oncological surgeon Heinrich Pophanken, M.D. Frau M.'s tumor, five centimeters (cm) in diameter, bulkier than a hen's egg, and situated inaccessibly on the pancreas, could not be removed even though a surgical incision had been made. Her case considered hopeless, with death expected within days, Dr. Pophanken merely closed the patient's incision without touching the tumor. He then asked Dr. Walter Kuhlmey to inject the woman with Polyerga® in order to ease her pain, lift fatigue, and stimulate a feeling of well-being.

Over four months with only minor interruptions, Dr. Kuhlmey administered to Frau M. three to six intramuscular injections per week of Polyerga®; and during the next two months he reduced the dosage to just two injections a week. Surprising everyone who knew the woman's circumstances, this treatment allowed her to live a good quality of life for three years longer than expected. She gained weight by restoration of her appetite, was cheerful during the entire period of convalescence, joined in family activities, and performed usual household chores as a wife and mother.

In June 1954, the patient fell ill with acute ileus, from which she died immediately after undergoing an operation to correct this new condition. At the autopsy, no more tumor tissue of any kind was found. Her pancreatic cancer had resolved, leaving no sign of its having been present except for extensive scarring on the organ. This serendipitous discovery was the beginning of cancer clinician Kuhlmey's looking at Polyerga® as a treatment for malignancies of all types.

Biochemical research was Dr. Walter Kuhlmey's primary interest, but he also taught medical students. In 1954, the Medical University of Madrid invited him to be visiting professor of biochemical medicine, and he remained in that position for four years. While the university provided a small stipend for his research, it was financially supported mainly by his wife's management of their company, HorFerVit Pharma GmbH (see page 38).

Two sons, Kristian and Jurgen, have participated with their father and mother to research and develop medical products against cancer. They built not only HorFerVit Pharma GmbH but also its sister production company, Idosan Pharma GmbH. Using sophisticated equipment, the trained scientific staff under the Kuhlmey family's supervision has turned out quality, safe, adjunctive, and supportive anticancer therapies. Their products take the form of organ extracts packaged as ampoules, tablets, and capsules, with the porcine spleen peptide formulation Polyerga® as their companies' major product.

Polyerga® Eliminates Rectal Cancer in a German Patient

Publishing in the German complementary and alternative medicine journal *Complementary Oncology Forum and Immunobiology Forum,* oncologist Klaus Maar, M.D., of Bieleseld, a suburban town in northern Germany, presented his patient's health history. An eighty-year-old former merchant seaman, Hans K., had become the victim of recurrent Stage II rectal cancer. Classified as a Dukes' B2 tumor, it extended through the bowel wall but had not spread to any lymph nodes. Herr K. consulted Dr. Maar just before Easter 1996 with symptoms typical of colorectal cancer: extensive rectal bleeding, constipation with long and narrow stools, abdominal pain, gas, vomiting, weight loss, and weakness.

Among other laboratory test readings, Herr K.'s immune system profile showed an extraordinarily low ratio of helper T-cells to suppressor T-cells. "His histological diagnosis was a differentiated tubular-growing adenocarcinoma of the rectum. This was the recurrence of a rectal carcinoma, which had been operated on September 9, 1993, for resection with end-to-end anastomosis," wrote Dr. Maar in his clinical journal report. "The patient was scheduled for hospital admission to undergo an operation fixed for that Monday after Easter. I attempted to convince Mr. K. that an operation was necessary, but he refused it and wished first to see if my biological treatment would be successful."

As it happens, 10 percent of all malignant tumors seen in the Western industrialized countries, including the United States and Germany, involve the colorectal region, with one-third of them occurring specifically in the rectum. Taken together, colon and rectal carcinoma are second only to lung cancer as a cause of cancer deaths.

About 90 percent of colorectal cancers come from polyps, pea-sized, mushroomlike growths protruding from the inner layer (mucosa) of the lower gastrointestinal tract. After surgery for removal of these polyps, recurrent cancer may be the ultimate cause of death in one-third of cases. And this was the likely situation for Hans K.

Because of his patient's definite refusal to undergo immediate surgery, Dr. Maar was forced into using a biological therapy adapted to fit the requirements of this former merchant seaman's immune system. The physician therefore commenced treatment using three particular therapies: daily ozone insufflation into the intestine, orally administered Wobe-Mugos® proteolytic enzymes, and subcutaneous injection of the Polyerga® immune stabilizer/biologic response modifier. Dr. Maar records that by itself, Polyerga® most effectively brought about cancer remission for Herr Hans K.

"In the middle of May 1996, I carried out a control rectoscopy and found that the tumour, which had been bigger than a plum, could not now be detected. Yet, a biopsy of the prior tumour had shown a medium grade, differentiated adenocarcinoma," Dr. Maar states. "My treatment was then continued for a further four weeks; afterward it was paused until the end of August.

"At the beginning of September 1996, a fourteen-day interval treatment in the form described was started again [but with the discontinuance of ozone insufflation and Wobe-Mugos® enzymes]. The patient always felt very fit and mentally balanced. I carried out the control rectoscopy again in October 1996, and it showed no tumour macroscopically. Furthermore, there was now also no neoplasm detectable histologically," says Dr. Maar. "No hyperplastic mucous membrane or indication of malignancy existed."

By July 1997, Hans K., having just turned eighty-two years old, felt so fit, youthful, and with a zest for life that he married again. Dr. Klaus Maar writes in his May 1999 CAM journal article, "Immune analyses of the patient taken during and after my Polyerga® treatment show a constant improvement and stabilization of his immune system."[1]

Ambulating Proof of Polyerga® Anti-Aging Attributes

The wife of Dr. Walter Kuhlmey exhibited her acumen as a dynamic businesswoman. The cost of medical research is exceedingly high, and her husband's focus was entirely on investigating all aspects of Polyerga® as a remedy for the prevention and treatment of degenerative diseases, especially cancer. Frau Grit Kuhlmey financed Dr. Walter Kuhlmey's efforts by turning their company into a highly profitable enterprise. She achieved success by dealing with domestic animal slaughterhouses, negotiating exclusive contracts, and trading in animal organs for pharmaceutical companies.

It was usual for Frau Kuhlmey to confirm organ viability by making visits directly to an abattoir, examining the freshly butchered organs, buying up quantities, setting prices for trades, and making deals for resale. This is one tough woman, who functioned effectively in a man's roughneck world and went on to accompany her husband to his lecture presentations, scientific conferences, medical meetings, and other conventions. All over the world, Frau Kuhlmey made contacts for Dr. Walter Kuhlmey. Believing totally in his work, she held discussions with authorities in the areas of diabetes, cancer, immune system suppression, and other degenerative diseases as they related to the administration of Polyerga®.

I accompanied Dr. Kristian Kuhlmey to his mother's tastefully furnished home in Oldenburg, Germany, and he rang her bell. After we identified ourselves over her intercom speaker system, Frau Kuhlmey sent the elevator down to fetch us and simultaneously ran down the three flights of stairs. She beat the elevator, which she never rides, simply because she requires the exercise. "Descending and ascending actual stairs is better for me than using my Stairmaster," she says. Her son and I stepped into the elevator and ascended, but before we could disembark at her apartment door, the lady had already arrived there to greet us.

What is the secret of her youthfulness? "For the past thirty-two years, one tablet a day of 100 mg of Polyerga® is the only nutritional supplement I have taken," states Frau Grit Kuhlmey, "and it prevents me from ever having illness of any kind."

Polyerga® Combined with Hyperthermia Causes Cancer Remission

In Wilhelmshaven, Germany, at the Gisunt Klinik for Complementary Medicine, a division of the Gisunt Institute for Preventive and Aesthetic Medicine, Polyerga® intramuscular (IM) and subcutaneous (SC) injections have been shown to react well against malignant tumors when such injections are combined with whole body hyperthermia (WBH). Adjunctively administered with the IM or SC Polyerga™ and combined with WBH, Polyerga Plus™ tablets and/or capsules assist in bringing about the remission of many cancerous types. The renowned German oncologist Holger Wehner, M.D., medical director of the Gisunt Klinik, reports that during the ten years of his utilizing these therapies together, he has never encountered any treatment side effects or contraindications. At least one new cancer patient daily who comes to receive his treatment program is administered Dr. Wehner's combination treatment program at his health-care facility.

In his systemic cancer multistep therapy (sCMT), Dr. Wehner applies a transfer of energy with infrared radiation which uses water filtration at a focal point of radiated heat consisting of 760 nanometers (nm) to 1,400 nm. This optimal amount of infrared radiation for the shrinkage of tumor tissue penetrates deep into the skin up to the capillary area of the corium (the underlying skin layer). It permits a rapid rise of body-core temperature and a high thermal constancy. Cancer cells respond adversely to the application of heat, especially to temperatures ranging near 42°C (108°F).

"What all types of infrared hyperthermia equipment have in common is that they induce a warming-up of the body over the skin," writes Dr. Wehner. "According to the laws of thermodynamics, there is no area of the body's interior, and no tumor, which is not affected by such a warming of the outer body shell. . . . During the hyperthermia treatment, the unclothed patient lies on the net of IRATHERM®2000 (the oven-like heating unit), and is warmed from above by two sets and from below by three sets of special lamps. Reflecting transparent foils hanging from the sides close off the warming area from draughts of air while the patient's head remains outside this area during the treatment. The warming of the patient can be controlled by varying the lamp power; moreover, the sets of lamps are individually adjustable."[2]

The systemic cancer multistep therapy was learned by Dr. Holger Wehner under a preceptorship he took with Manfred von Ardenne, M.D., at the Von Ardenne Institute of Applied Medical Research GmbH in Dresden, Germany. Dr. Von Ardenne had used the sCMT from 1989 onward as an effective complementary/alternative treatment for those patients with recurrent cancer who had failed to respond to accepted conventional cancer therapies. The sCMT involves the concurrent application of the synergistically acting steps of three particular physiological effects: an extreme whole body hyperthermia, an induced hyperglycemia, and a relative hyperoxemia.[3]

Extreme WBH operates with a hyperthermia dose of 42.0°C to 42.3°C body-core temperature applied over sixty to ninety minutes. It serves for producing the effect of thermal carcinolysis (the breaking down of cancer cells), the selective inhibition of the microcirculation in cancer tissue, and the intensification of its selective acidification by hyperglycemia.[4]

Induced hyperglycemia causes a selective stimulation of the aerobic glycolytic metabolism of cancer cells discovered in 1924 by German biochemist Otto Warburg, Ph.D., M.D. Dr. Warburg's investigation of the metabolism of cancer cells led him to the view, which was subsequently confirmed, that cancer cells exist in the body as facultative anaerobes, capable of growth without oxygen, whereas the normal body cells are obligate aerobes, incapable of anaerobic growth. This discovery was expected to have far-reaching results in aiding the understanding of—and ability to control—neoplastic growth. It has![5]

Glycolytic cancer cells become overacidified so that the cancer cell's membranes and the membranes of its cellular organelles become damaged. There is then a selective increase in the thermosensitization of cancer cells by about 1.5°C and, in addition, an increase in its radiosensitization by a factor of 2.5. Enhanced effectiveness of simultaneously applied cytotoxic anticancer drugs occurs as well.[6]

Because the temperature of 42°C alone is insufficient to cause an adequate damaging of cancer cells, the simultaneously administered Polyerga® becomes vitally important, for the combination of heat and porcine spleen hormonal components work to the cancer's great disadvantage. Futhermore, the strong increase in blood glucose levels during the extreme hyperthermia phase concurrently contribute to a maintained hemodynamic and respiratory sufficiency.[7]

The highly selective lysosomal cytolysis chain reaction which takes place in the acidic milieu or under sCMT conditions contributes to therapeutic cancer cell damage. Selective inhibition of microcirculation in cancer tissue is promoted by its overacidification. Cancer cells starve to death from undergoing a lack of blood supply.[8]

Relative hyperoxemia is implemented by the controlled oxygenation of the patient's inspired air during the extreme hyperthermia phase.[9]

On April 21, 2001, I visited the Gisunt Klinik and tape-recorded an extensive interview with Dr. Holger Wehner. At that time he declared: "Among cancer patients taking treatment here at the

Gisunt Klinik, 99 percent do experience some improvement in their symptoms. It's rare that any individual might report not feeling or functioning better. For nearly all patients, the quality of life is better by our administering integrative holistic therapies.

"Alone, as the sole cancer treatment, Polyerga® in the form of a self-administered SC injection administered into the abdominal skin, or in the form of an IM injection given into the butt and taken once daily, is excellent anticancer therapy. Alternatively, Polyerga® swallowed as three tablets of Polyerga Plus™ once a day before breakfast works well too. This porcine spleen extract by itself brings about a five-year survival with incomplete cancer remission overall for 60 percent of my patients," said the oncologist from Wilhelmshaven, Germany. "Since the variety of cancer therapies are quite costly which some patients cannot afford, my prescribing injective Polyerga® or the tablets of Polyerga Plus™ is a good stopgap measure.

"Using Polyerga® not as the sole treatment but as adjunctive therapy with hyperthermia, I invariably find that the patient's result is improved markedly. Again, at this clinic, using the combined therapy, 80 percent of our patients undergo five-year survival from experiencing cancer remission," Dr. Holger Wehner stated. "Unlike conventional cancer chemotherapy which directly attacks cancer cells, holistic type oncologists in Germany work to elevate the action of a patient's immune system. My belief is that most important for any cancer patient is to receive treatment that boosts the body's immunity. Polyerga® and whole body hyperthermia in combination achieve such a boost very well."

Resources

Dr. Holger Wehner's Gisunt Klinik is located in an extreme northern part of Germany, Wilhelmshaven, on a stretch of coast abutting the North Sea. Public transportation is not readily available. Oncologist Holger Wehner, M.D., who speaks some English but requires his daughter to interpret, offers more specific information about his use of Polyerga® and hyperthermia.

Reach Dr. Holger Wehner at the Gisunt Klinik fuer Komplementaere Medizin, a division of the Gisunt Institut fuer Praeventive und Aesthetische Medizin, Muehlenweg 144, D-26384 Wilhelmshaven, Germany; telephone 011(49)4421-75566-0; fax 011(49)4421-75566-10; website http://www.gisunt.de or (another website) http://www.comedverlag.de.

PART TWO

Carnivora®

This section has been written as the result of
numerous personal consultations with
German oncologist Helmut G. Keller, M.D.

3

Cancer Remission Rates of Carnivora®

Formerly practicing as a nutritional therapist in Westport, Connecticut, tall, blond, and attractive, forty-one-year-old Stephanie V., N.D., a native of the Netherlands, in February 1994, discovered what she describes as "a fairly large lump in my right breast. I was worried," she says.

"Diagnostic procedures I underwent, using both mammography and ultrasound, were negative. But the biopsy performed for me by a Bridgeport surgeon denied that the lump was benign. Instead the biopsy showed my breast was invaded by a malignancy, an intraductal adenocarcinoma one and one-half centimeters in diameter," Dr. V. recounts. "The finding was surprising to both the surgeon and me, since I had gone through two separate breast examinations during November 1993 with no pathology reported. So my doctor determined that this was an aggressively malignant tumor growing excessively fast. And a lumpectomy was needed.

"After excision left clean borders, the surgeon recommended radiation to my breast. I didn't opt for that but instead flew to Bad Steben, Germany, to take treatment from oncologist Dr. Helmut G. Keller. [Dr. Keller has since moved his oncology practice out of Germany.] I knew Dr. Keller from having met him a few times while attending international medical meetings and sci-

entific conferences. He is a kind, concerned, renowned physician and the discoverer of the Venus' flytrap extract Carnivora®,"
says Dr. V. "Inasmuch as I'm well informed about German alternative cancer treatments—having referred American patients to
that country's clinics frequently—I was particularly impressed
with results achieved by Dr. Keller. *[Author's note: Helmut G.
Keller, M.D., of Nordhalben, Germany, is a primary oncological consultant source for information offered in this book.]*

"I was treated for four weeks at Dr. Keller's clinic with intravenous (IV) Carnivora®," continues the Westport nutritionist.
"Also, because my tumor was growing so aggressively, Dr.
Keller gave me additional therapy with whole body hyperthermia, interferon injections, and hydrazine sulfate. Back home,
since my T-cells were not yet returned to a normal level, I kept
up the Carnivora® infusions for four weeks more. With help
from a friend who injected me, I administered the IV Carni-
vora® to myself every day.

"When my blood tests showed themselves as normal, I went
on a routine six-month program of taking intramuscular (IM)
injections using Carnivora®. There, too, I faithfully continued to
inject myself. At the conclusion of the series of IM injections, I
began myself on the oral administration of Carnivora® at a
dosage of forty drops in four ounces of purified water swallowed three times a day. This procedure has kept me in permanent breast cancer remission for over seven and a half years,"
affirms Dr. V. "Of course, I keep an eye on my prior symptoms,
which I believe are eliminated completely, by checkups for
them that I undergo with a range of blood tests. The tests include some sophisticated tumor markers, and checking counts
for the normality of white blood cells, the natural killer cells,
T-lymphocytes, B-lymphocytes, the various subpopulations related to the helper-suppressor ratio, and much more.

"I use the popular test being performed in Germany that I
had learned from Dr. Keller—the lipid-associated sialic acid in
plasma (LASA-P) tumor biomarker," Dr. V. says. "Every three

months I send my blood to be studied by another German physician who practices in the United States, Dietmar Schild-wachter, M.D., at his laboratory, the Southern Consultants International, Inc. Dr. Schildwachter determines my immune status by performing a full cancer profile, including the DHEA test and more tumor markers. *[Note: Please see the Resources section at the conclusion of this chapter to acquire addresses and telephone numbers for those health professionals and products cited herein.]*

"All cancer markers have been turning up normal for me. My immune system is fine—behaving appropriately—and only varies up and down according to the stress that I experience during daily practice and usual living. I'm doing well," declares Dr. V. "But I haven't personally shared my cancer remission story with any of my patients as yet. You see, I'm writing a book on the subject, and I wish to have the privilege of revealing my own good fortune sometime in the future."

Chemotherapy Endangers Another
Connecticut Resident

Adrienne R., a wife, mother, and massage therapist working out of her home in my own city of Stamford, Connecticut, in September 1985, at age forty-one, was diagnosed with cancer from biopsies of her left supraclavicular and right inguinal area lymph nodes. Conventional oncological treatment options were offered to the patient (six months of chemotherapy followed by three months of radiation); instead, she elected to follow a macrobiotic diet to control her non-Hodgkin's, nondisseminated lymphocytic lymphoma (lymphosarcoma). Microscopic sections of the tumors were further described by a pathologist as poorly differentiated and of the nodular type. Also a bone marrow aspirate showed lymphocytosis.

Macrobiotics served Mrs. R. well until some tumors reappeared in her left inguinal region. She took eleven locally applied radiotherapies, and the tumors disappeared. A respected oncologist in New York City persuaded her to follow up with a course of chemotherapy for several months using the single cytotoxic agent cyclophosphamide (Cytoxan™). During our interview, she told me it did not help much.

Then Mrs. R. was treated with a double combination of cytotoxics, vinblastine (Velban™) and cyclophosphamide, from August to October 1989, and a little later melphalan (Alkeran™) was added to the combination but with no response. Next, she again received intravenous cyclophosphamide alone. These treatments may have made her tumor burden more comfortable, but they did nothing to take away the generalized cancer, which lingered.

In another year, she underwent a course of radiotherapy with 2,000 centigray (cGy) to the right groin. With all of these toxic cancer treatments being applied, Mrs. R. remained faithful to her macrobiotic program of eating and found that she was most helped by her avoidance of sugar.

In December 1992 her legs became swollen because of lymphatic blockage from tumors. Following her doctors' advice, Mrs. R. took more chemotherapy, six cycles with cyclophosphamide, prednisone, and the antibiotic derivative doxorubicin hydrochloride (Adriamycin™),[1] for a total dose of 285 mg/m^2. The treatment continued until April 19, 1993, when some tumors disappeared. But then they did return within one year of her finishing the chemotherapy.

Adriamycin™ produces severely adverse side effects for the heart in 11 percent of patients who receive this cytotoxic agent. In eight out of nine patients given doses greater than 300 mg/m^2 of body surface area, decreased left ventricular function takes place. When patients take a total dose greater than 500 mg/m^2, 30 percent of them develop cardiac failure. Although she received less than a total toxic dose, this severe heart dysfunction happened to Adrienne R. Perhaps it was because she also had previously been administered cyclophosphamide, inasmuch as doses between 60 and 120 mg/kg of this drug are responsible for heart muscle death or heart attacks.[2]

With Cancer in Remission, Cardiomyopathy Strikes Mrs. R.

In June 1994, Mrs. R. developed an upper respiratory tract illness diagnosed as pneumonia. When she failed to improve with antibiotics, her doctors decided she actually was suffering from congestive heart failure. Diagnosis by means of an echocardiogram showed that the patient had an ejection fraction of between 20 and 25 percent—exceedingly low. She was considered to have developed cardiomyopathy from having received Adriamycin™ and associated cytotoxic drugs. Owing to severe pleural effusion and symptoms of heart failure, the patient became a semi-invalid with restricted activities. She no longer could play tennis, which was her passion.

Mrs. R.'s poorly differentiated lymphocytic lymphoma of the nodular type returned with a vengeance so that she was forced to consult oncologists, pathologists, biopsy surgeons, and other medical specialists repeatedly from January 9 to April 10, 1995. Cancerous masses appeared in both breasts, on her neck, in the cervical, axillary, and inguinal areas, and then around the eye sockets as multiple periorbital nodules.

Mrs. R. refused further toxic therapies recommended by physicians, and a month later she traveled to Bad Steben to receive IV Carnivora® daily from Dr. Keller. As a result of the infusions, her nodules and tumors did not enlarge or spread but steadily grew smaller. Some disappeared. Then the patient returned home for a few months, but swelling of the right leg from cardiomyopathy started up. At home, she received physiotherapy and oxygen therapy from technicians.

Because tumors were reappearing, she returned to Bad Steben in November 1995. Since IV Carnivora® was hard on her veins, she briefly flew back to the United States for insertion of a portacath (which did not work) and then went back to Germany for more treatment until March 1996. Another portacath inserted in a German hospital worked just fine and she received more IV Carnivora®. The cancerous lumps grew smaller and disappeared.

During her return flight to the United States, Mrs. R. could hardly breathe because of fluid accumulated in the right chest cavity, and her heart felt like it "blew up balloon-size." Now it was the complicating cardiomyopathy that endangered her life. She took injections into the pleural space, and investigated having a chest tube inserted for sclerosis.

Despite the atmospheric pressures of an airline cabin being difficult on her heart, in September 1996 she flew back to Dr. Keller's clinic because some new lumps had appeared. This time the oncological researcher and clinician administered Carnivora® to Mrs. R. by means of a new portable pump he had developed. The tumors went away. She returned home outfitted with the pump and a supply of Carnivora® which kept her cancer in remission, where it remained.

Computerized tomography (CT) of Mrs. R.'s chest showed a very large right pleural effusion, a moderate left pleural effusion, and mediastinal adenopathy. The abdominal CT showed extensive para-aortic adenopathy. Her life was in danger from the cardiomyopathy.

With all of her tumor markers and other tests showing up negative for evidence of non-Hodgkin's lymphoma, on December 15, 1996, Dr. Keller advised Mrs. R. to discontinue using the Carnivora® pump; besides, her heart could no longer tolerate the heart muscle stress it created.

While she remained in cancer remission, the conventional chemotherapy and other toxic therapies that she received in the

United States overburdened this loving wife and mother with severe congestive heart failure. The heart problem was confirmed by her conventionally practicing American doctors as arising from Adriamycin™. They said it had brought on cardiomyopathy. Heart failure became Adrienne R.'s single life-threatening illness, and on May 17, 1998, it killed her. Carnivora® had prevented her from dying of cancer.

"Toxic Cancer Therapies Do More Patient Harm Than Good"

"If physicians prescribing for patients diagnosed with malignancies would begin immediately to use biological, natural, and nontoxic treatments, the worldwide medical community would have much greater success in achieving cancer remissions and/or cures. However, we who dispense nontoxic therapies most often must confront cancer in its end stages," emphasizes Helmut G. Keller, M.D. "After immune abilities have been ruined by chemotherapy or radiation, is when cancer patients find their way to nontoxic therapies as a last resort. And usually they come not as a result of physician referral but rather on their own. Holistic oncologists fighting to save lives this way are being presented with impossible odds!

"It's a known fact—even the American Cancer Society admits it—that a mere 5 percent of cancers are cured by chemotherapy. So how can those doctors who practice conventional oncology be so self-satisfied with their dubious accomplishments?" asks Dr. Keller. "They are traveling down the wrong road to a dead end with their patients ending dead! These sick people turn to the medical profession for lifesaving help but don't find any. Still, there's a physiological answer that's been overlooked these many decades.

"Nontoxic cancer therapies alternative to the present poisonous and inadequate treatment methods utilize a patient's immunological self-defense system. Nontoxic cancer therapies regenerate immunity and readily kill off multimillions of tumor cells. This happens not out of neglect or abuse of one's immune system but by its being nurtured, bolstered, and reinforced," Dr. Keller says. "Immune system stimulation is mandatory in our modern polluted environments.

"For patients with early malignancies who come to me for treatment before undergoing any noxious therapies, I achieve cancer remission for almost 98 percent of them," states Dr. Keller. "As long as a patient's malignant tumor ranges in the microsize area—below 10^9 malignant cells (pinpoint size)—my statistical patient records indicate something near to a 98 percent rate of remission. The only problem I face is that very few people with cancer seek out uninjurious therapies prior to trying and failing with highly toxic chemotherapy, radiation therapy, or both.

"The current treatment procedure for malignancies should be turned on its head, with cancer patients trying harmless therapies first. Only if nonhurtful care fails them might the patient accept the risk of cytotoxins because they may offer some small chance to stay alive for a little while. Cancer is curable but not with chemotherapy or radiation. Toxic cancer therapies do much more patient harm than good and should be avoided, if possible," Dr. Keller affirms.

Conventional oncological practices that employ cytotoxic agents are killing off the most important organ of an ill person, the immune system. If they could be weighed collectively, the immune-competent cells of the human body would come up to 1.5 kilograms (kg). Toxic compounds with such generic names as doxorubicin, fluorouracil, methotrexate, cyclophosphamide, cisplatin, vincristine, vinblastine, agent orange, and two dozen others annhilate the immune-competent cells. "All of these drugs have one characteristic in common," writes Ralph W. Moss, Ph.D., "they are poisonous. They work because they're poisons."[3]

Long-Term Exposure to Carnivora® Obliterates Cancer Cells

Studies of Carnivora® were conducted by Professor Dieter Kurt Todorov, M.D., Ph.D., D.Sc., chief of the Laboratories of Oncopharmacology at the National Oncological Center of Bulgaria. Half of each year he works in Bulgaria and the other half he spends in cancer research at Heidelberg University in Heidelberg, Germany. From a series of seven unpublished reports on his German investigations, Professor Todorov advised Dr. Keller that cancer cells subjected to long-term exposure with Carnivora® are either considerably reduced in number or completely obliterated. The findings that follow are based on this cancer pharmacologist's laboratory observations:

• Study One. In his first study, Professor Todorov learned that ovarian cancer cells in a rat model tumor (in vivo) exposed to 200 nanograms (ng) per milliliter (ml) of Carnivora® reduced their number from 1,500 cells to 435 cells within forty-eight hours of exposure.

• Study Two. Professor Todorov's second study carried out for seven days on human glioblastoma (brain cancer) cells saw 200 ng/ml of Carnivora® diminish the cancer cell number by half (from exactly 109 cells to 55). He proved that the smaller a tumor is, the more effectively Carnivora® works to bring about reduction in separate cellular units. For this reason, it's imperative to administer the pressed juice of Venus' flytrap to patients as soon as any size, shape, or type of cancer is discovered.

If the cancer cells composed of the actual tumor number 10^6 or less, the patient's malignancy is reversible and curable. With the cancer cell number rising to 10^9 or higher, however, cure is not possible. Between these two levels of cell content in a malignancy, reversibility and curability is variable depending on the patient's immune system competency and the cancer's aggressiveness. Dr. Keller says, "If you catch the cancer too late, it runs away to kill the patient."

A surgeon who skillfully reduces the patient's tumor burden can improve odds for survival to as high as 30 percent; nevertheless, the chance of cancer metastasis still remains at around 70 percent. A primary lesson to be learned here is that the point of no return must be avoided by treating microsize cancer growths with Carnivora® as an immediate therapeutic action.

• Study Three. With his third investigation, Professor Todorov exposed 2,500 experimental human sarcoma cells to Carnivora® for seventy-two hours, at which time they dropped in number to 880 cells. This in vitro experiment can be transposed into an in vivo finding.

• Study Four. In the next experiment, Professor Todorov reported that 1,711 cells of human ovarian cancer diminished to 359 cells upon being exposed to 200 ng/ml of Carnivora® during a forty-eight-hour period. This particular cancer failed to respond to chemotherapy with cisplatin. Despite the ovarian cancer cells being chemotherapy resistant, Carnivora® was able to reduce the cell number.

• Study Five. In Professor Todorov's fifth study, he examined cancer cells on a petri dish and then under the microscope. The professor showed that treatment with 200 ng/ml of Carnivora® reduced 3,100 cells of human T-lymphoblastic leukemia to 1,820 cancer cells in seventy-two hours. This is laboratory proof of Dr. Keller's experience in clinical practice that Carnivora® works well after its long exposure (from four weeks up to six months) to the blood constituents of chronic myeloid leukemia and chronic lymphatic leukemia. Such long exposure of weeks or months is possible by application of a small and convenient-to-use pump developed by Dr. Keller. (The full description of this Carnivora® pump is presented below.)

Based on Dr. Keller's prolonged period of experience with treating leukemias using his Carnivora® pump, these blood dyscrasias may be considered reversible and curable. All of the leukemia patients who have consulted him during the past year are still alive, reside in their own homes, or ambulate as tourists vacationing in Germany. They have the pump attached to their belts while projecting a catheter into an arm and remain in treatment with blood drawn regularly for examination.

Confirming Dr. Keller's declaration that he is achieving remission of cancer for almost 98 percent of patients who don't take cytotoxic therapies, I must offer the following report based on my observations as a medical journalist: Most of those patients receiving Carnivora™ but who have undergone *no* chemotherapy or radiation are thriving; those who have received either or both of the described cytotoxins are not in such good condition.

- Study Six. From results of the sixth study, Professor Todorov was able to contradict Dr. Keller's prior belief that Carnivora® does not work against sarcoma. The oncological pharmacologist from Bulgaria took 2,200 multidrug-resistant human sarcoma cells and reduced them to 1,130 cells in seventy-two hours by exposing them to 400 mg of Carnivora®. As a result of this new finding, Dr. Keller treated patients with microsize sarcoma tumors with Carnivora®, and they became well by becoming free of cancer. Cure of sarcoma occurs after long-term exposure to Carnivora®.

Dr. Keller advises that in the case of microsize sarcomatous tumors being present, the patients' LASA-P tumor markers will invariably be elevated. The LASA-P® (lipid-associated sialic acid in plasma) test is a biomarker, useful in a wide range of malignancies. The LASA-P test reflects alteration in the surface membrane of malignant cells and measures total gangliosides and glycoproteins by the biochemical extraction and partition method developed by Dr. N. Katopodis et al. Sensitivities range between 77 percent and 97 percent, depending on cell of origin of the neoplasm. Studies have shown improved predictive value when the LASA-P test is combined with other biomarkers in biomarker profiles. The LASA-P test is described in more detail in this book's final chapter.

• Study Seven. The seventh investigation conducted by Professor Todorov involved his exposing human leukemia cells—all of which had proven to be multidrug-resistant—to 200 ng/ml Carnivora®. Within seventy-two hours, the abnormal, immature, and leukemic white blood cells responded well to Carnivora® and were reduced in number from 2,250 to 570. Leukemia is successfully treated with this squeezed juice of the Venus' flytrap.

The Criminality of Conventional Cytotoxic Cancer Therapies

To illustrate how cytotoxic cancer therapies do serious damage to patients, if they live a while after taking them, Dr. Helmut Keller tells us about Maureen, a young woman from Ireland who underwent radiation therapy and came away with an ugly, debilitating, chronic unilateral lymphedema of the left arm. In rendering an opinion about the stupidity or criminality connected with using toxic cancer therapies, what happened to this young woman speaks volumes. Her arms swelled to triple size with lymphedema, all her hair fell out, and she vomited many times daily for four weeks until she died from cytotoxicity from the radiation.

Because of his strong desire to offer a place of comfort and care for patients with malignancies, Dr. Keller is rendering his oncological services in a medically free environment offshore from the United States. A great number of his patients have been Americans and Canadians. Many more cancer clinics, which provide patients with complementary and alternative therapies, are locating offshore because people have recognized the failure of conventionally rendered chemotherapy and radiation therapy. Dr. Helmut Keller has established his cancer clinic dedicated to the treatment of degenerative diseases with fully staffed departments focusing on psychoneuroimmunology, oncology, neurology, Carnivora® therapy, hyperthermia, urology, and interdisciplinary medicine.

Consulting with the staff and patients numerous times each month, Dr. Keller is medical director and president of the clinic. He also continues to be in charge of daily treatment strategies for patients.

A Full Description of the Phytonutrient Carnivora®

Carnivora® is the processed and purified juice (production patent pending) taken from the Venus' flytrap plant. The digestive juice of this plant is a phytonutrient that attacks and destroys every variety of cellular malignancy and is especially effective on primitive cancer tumor tissues as opposed to highly differentiated ones. Nevertheless, because of Carnivora's® ability to modulate and stimulate the immune system of both humans and animals, its use is indicated for all types of malignancies, including carcinomas, sarcomas, blood dyscrasias (the leukemias), and most definitely cancer metastases. It's beneficial as treatment for some of the other degenerative diseases as well.

Carnivora® also acts advantageously as a growth inhibitor of the human immunodeficiency virus (HIV) and for moderating those more severe symptoms occurring in acquired immunode-ficiency syndrome (AIDS).

For cancers affecting the brain, and those that have a ten-dency to spread to the brain and the central nervous system, Carnivora® is diluted in 20 percent mannitol. Mannitol is a sugar that opens the blood-brain barrier and tends to concen-trate Carnivora® solution in the brain. An additional and desir-able effect is that it acts to drain the edema from this compressed and sensitive area.

The Portable Carnivora® Systemic Pump

Carnivora® may be taken orally as drops and capsules. Its equally refined injectable form works well intravenously and subcutaneously; however, the ideal Carnivora® treatment is ad-ministered systemically by means of a mechanical pump the size of a portable Walkman cassette player.

The portable, systemic pumping device—hooked onto a belt at the waist or hanging from a chain around the neck—contains the Carnivora® injectable solution supplied in a plastic bag. The bag containing Venus' flytrap juice is replaced every seven to ten days. A tube from the bag attaches to the input of a central venous catheter or subcutaneous portacath. Closing its lid winds up and starts the pump, which begins a moderate flow of 0.6 cubic centimeters (cc) of the Venus' flytrap solution into a vein in the body for twenty-four hours a day, seven days a week. The pumped solution should be used for a period of one to three months or longer, as required.

The dosage for a standard intravenous infusion is 5 cc of Carnivora® diluted in 250 cc of 0.9 percent sodium chloride or in 250 cc of 20 percent mannitol. If not using the portable sys-temic pump, the patient receives an IV infusion over a three- to four-hour time span in the morning. Adjunctive to the IV infusion, a 1-cc subcutaneous injection of Carnivora® is advantageous as well, to be self-administered in the evening in order to maintain the twenty-four-hour influence.

After three to six months of initial treatment, the malignant tumors usually stop growing and decrease in size. Then cancer reversal takes place when two subcutaneous Carnivora® injections of just 1 cc each are taken, one in the morning and one in the evening. It's appropriate for these injections to be accompanied by the oral intake five times daily of fifty drops of Carnivora® diluted in purified water. Or two of the Carnivora® capsules may be substituted for the drops. To overcome a life-threatening disease, up to six capsules should be taken daily. Oral administration should occur before meals or on an empty stomach and continue for a period of approximately two years.

Until a few years ago, 2 cc of the highly refined Carnivora® (which was utilized by Dr. Stephanie V., as described at the opening of this chapter) often was self-administered every other day as an intramuscular injection, but that method has now been abandoned. IM injections are less useful than other administration techniques, and they could cause the rise of uncomfortable inflamed bumps or knots in the buttocks.

Cancer of the urinary bladder is well served by injecting 5 cc of the pure Carnivora® into this organ three times weekly.

Pleural and abdominal effusion is best treated by removing the accumulated fluid and inserting 5 cc of Carnivora® in its stead.

Cervical cancer responds well to Carnivora® when the tip of a tampon is soaked with the solution and the wet tampon is placed deep in the vagina. The patient should do this before bedtime.

Lung cancer will show marked improvement by having the patient inhale Carnivora® drops three to five times per day using a cold steam vaporizer without ultrasound. Each inhalation should include 2 cc of sodium chloride.

Carnivora® is compatible with all known nontoxic treatments and may be employed in combination with any of them. Robert C. Atkins, M.D., medical director of the Atkins Center in New York City, employs Carnivora® as part of his generalized model for cancer treatment. He is impressed mightily by the results achieved when the remedy is used. "The reason these results are impressive is that they show that the treatment 'works' and is suitable to act as an effective partner to other nontoxic treatments that also work," Dr. Atkins states. "Carnivora® may work in a different way from other therapies, by rendering the tumor less malignant rather than by destroying any tissue."[4]

Beware of Fraudulent Carnivora®

Having been told the therapeutic applications and best methods of delivering the patent pending, trade name registered Venus' flytrap solution, now you're offered a warning: Avoid the imitations of Carnivora® which are not produced under the strict refining process developed by Helmut G. Keller, M.D. There are a few of these imitations around which are trading on the reputation of Dr. Keller's original manufacturing company.

The practices of imitators are exceedingly dangerous rip-offs for the end users, who ingest assorted poisons and antigens. Remember from whence the Venus' flytrap gets its name. This plant captures and digests flies, worms, mosquitoes, roaches, and other assorted bugs with all of their associated impurities.

Mrs. Ann L. of Falls Church, Virginia, wrote to me advising: "Thank you so much for validating my concern about the [imitation] extract I recently purchased for my husband, Jan. He had Lyme disease. Fortunately we were aware enough to stop the ingestion of this fradulent extract. Jan just started feeling *worse* after three days of taking one-quarter teaspoonful three times per day!"

Using his electrodermal screening machine, naturopath Marvin Schweitzer, N.D., of Norwalk, Connecticut, tested two American-made Carnivora® knockoffs that he stocked in his dispensary. He checked these two brands of drops against Dr. Keller's Carnivora® oral solution. The Keller drops had been brought to Dr. Schweitzer by his patient Adrienne R. of Stamford, Connecticut, whom I have already described.

"That day, on this patient, electroacupuncture according to Voll (EAV) tested compatibility to see if the three substances labeled as Carnivora® balanced meridians. In Adrienne's case, Dr. Keller's Carnivora® tested strongly, positively, and solidly but not the other two Venus' flytrap substances," Dr. Schweitzer says. "There were differences with the American-made products which, according to my machine's computerized ohm meter, were not advantageous for this patient. It was an objective reading, for I'm not prejudiced in any way about the Venus' flytrap solutions. I have no axe to grind."

Research turns up at least six imitations of Carnivora®. My suggestion is unambiguous. Any dispensing or prescribing health professional should be cautious about which Venus' flytrap product is recommended for patients' applications.

Resources

To receive further information about tumor biomarkers and/or cancer profiles from Dietmar Schildwachter, M.D., contact him at his laboratory or commercial firm, Southern Consultants International, Inc., P.O. Box 16602, Dulles International Airport, Washington, D.C. 20041; telephone (703) 430-7789; fax (703) 430-8189.

Also become informed about other cancer marker tests used by German oncologists that I describe in the final chapter of this book.

To receive more complete information about the natural and

nontoxic alternative cancer therapies provided at the clinic just offshore from the United States newly established by Dr. Helmut G. Keller, M.D., telephone owner, president, and CEO of Carnivora Research, Inc., Richard Ostrow, toll free within the United States at (866) 836-8735 or call from outside the U.S.A. at 001-(727) 781-0162.

Or e-mail Richard Ostrow at his manufacturer/distributor's commercial e-mail address: carnivora2000@yahoo.com.

Or you may reach Dr. Helmut Keller for personal medical information at another e-mail address which reaches him anywhere he is traveling in the world. It is: doc h keller@yahoo.com.

Although it is best to communicate with him by e-mail, the home base for Helmut Keller, M.D., is Nikolaus-Feulner Strasse 22, D-96365 Nordhalben, Germany; telephone 011-49-9267-1702; fax 011-49-9267-1708.

The processed and purified Carnivora® pressed juice in the form of oral drops is approved for dispensing to patients and doctors by the German Health Authority (Germany's food and drug administration) known as *B farm* (previously called *Bundesgesundheitamt* or BGA). Carnivora® in its intravenous, intramuscular, and subcutaneous injectable forms are available by prescription from Dr. Keller.

Carnivora® may be acquired for cancer prevention, maintenance, and/or treatment as self-administered capsules and/or extract as liquid drops by purchase from the manufacturer/distributor. To order, contact Richard Ostrow, president and chief executive officer (CEO) of Carnivora Research, Inc.; use the same telephone numbers as previously indicated. You may reach Richard Ostrow from overseas at 001-(727) 781-0162 or call toll free from anywhere in the United States to (866) 836-8735 (866 VENUS FLY).

The Carnivora® injectable solution awaits approval from *B farm* but may be available to some patients under the German FDA rules when Dr. Keller acts as the prescribing physician.

Because of variables in legal regulations, sometimes the purified juice of Venus' flytrap can be obtained by other licensed physicians directly from Dr. Helmut Keller. Telephone or e-mail to the product's manufacturer/distributor or e-mail to the physician/discoverer himself to learn why, how much, when, and answers to other questions about Carnivora®.

4

Cancer-Killing Components in Carnivora®

During a lecture he gave in 1875, directly after publishing one of his major scientific works, *Insectivorous Plants*,[1] the author of *On the Origin of Species by Means of Natural Selection*, English naturalist Charles Robert Darwin, stated: "The Venus-flytrap, *Dionaea muscipula*, is the most wonderful plant in the world."

Charles Darwin's statement is true not only because of the plant's behavior but also as a result of its medicinal value for humans and other animals. The pressed juice of *Dionaea muscipula* eliminates nearly all microbial infections and approximately 98 percent of the time reverses various types of microsize malignancies (in which the tumor's cellular number ranges from 10^6 to 10^9 [one million to ten thousand million] cells). This remission of small cancers occurs when application of refined Venus' flytrap juice known commercially as Carnivora® is accompanied by specific natural, nontoxic remedies and the patient has avoided chemotherapy, radiation therapy, and/or auxiliary cytotoxic agents. Carnivora® together with other nontoxic therapies is far superior for cancer treatment to either chemotherapy or radiation therapy or the combination of chemotherapy and radiation.

What I've written here is restricted only by the stipulation that the carnivorous plant's pressed juice must be purified to the highest degree so as to eliminate any antigenic proteins ingested by the Venus' flytrap. For therapeutic application, the substance must show less than 0.5 nanograms per milliliter (ng/ml) of endotoxin activity.

This purity is accomplished by use of a patented production process now belonging worldwide to Carnivora Research, Inc. From my journalistic investigations of it over a fourteen-year period, Carnivora® fits the description of highest purity for the pressed juice of Venus' flytrap. I base my stated conviction on four particular circumstances:

1. the experience of my wife, who successfully used the product and held off recurrence of her breast cancer from 1987 to 1999

2. discussions with a minimum of 300 people who had ingested Venus' flytrap juice

3. my evaluations of patient records furnished by those physicians administering refined Venus' flytrap juice

4. vast amounts of personal correspondence plus numerous interviews with the product's discoverer, Dr. Helmut Keller of Nordhalben, Germany.

A 50-milliliter (ml) bottle of Carnivora® contains the sterile pressed juice of the entire fresh plant, *Dionaea muscipula*, adjusted to 2 percent dry residue and isotonicity with mannitol. (Mannitol is a natural 6-carbon sugar alcohol formed by reduction of mannose or fructose, which is widely distributed in plants and fungi. It finds use in medicine as an osmotic diuretic in the prophylaxis of acute renal failure, in the evaluation of acute oliguria, and for reducing intraocular and cerebrospinal fluid pressure and volume.) Thus, 1 ml of Carnivora® contains *Dionaea muscipula* juice adjusted to 2 percent which totals 0.33 ml of residue, 0.33 ml of 86 percent ethanol, and aqua purificata (sterile water) 0.34 ml or 0.34 percent.

The Actual Therapeutic Ingredients in Venus' Flytrap Juice

Nature has provided us with numerous nutritional protective agents that support and enhance our immune systems. The best nutritional support we know of is Carnivora®, a phytonutrient product derived from the juice of the Venus' flytrap plant (*Dionaea muscipula*). Carnivora® supplements mimic the body's own defense agents and support a stronger immune reaction. The supplements, developed by Carnivora Research, Inc., maintain the carefully balanced immune system mechanisms. These mechanisms enhance the immune system response in persons suffering from poor health, and maintain optimum immune response in otherwise healthy persons who are suffering from stress, whether internal or external.

"In 1973, more than twenty-eight years ago, I discovered why the juice of Venus' flytrap is such an effective dietary supplement for the immune system. As you know, this plant is expert at trapping its own meals through a sensitive biological response process. When a fly or other small insect touches the delicate hairs of the plant's 'mouth,' it causes the mouth to close quickly, trapping the insect inside the plant," Dr. Helmut Keller explains. "Juicy liquids inside the plant's mouth are capable of digesting animal and vegetable materials. Interestingly, they do not digest the plant itself. From this observation, I have concluded that the Venus' flytrap must possess an advanced type of immune system capable of distinguishing between harmful intruder organisms and its own materials.

"In fact, the plant digests only the 'primitive,' undeveloped, undifferentiated cells of its prey. These 'primitive' cells are the same kind of cells that intrude into the human body as harmful bacteria, fungi, or which are overproduced due to stress, exposure to pollutants or poor dietary habits, and which the body's immune system is programmed to attack," continues Dr. Keller. Supplementing the diet with components of the Venus' flytrap juice supports the human immune system by fortifying the body's own defense mechanisms.

"As Darwin implied, the beauty and intelligence of this remarkable insect-eating plant cannot be overemphasized. It is one of nature's storehouses of phytonutrients for the human immune system," says Dr. Keller. "Over the past decade, Carnivora Research, Inc., the manufacturer/distributor with which I am associated, has refined the procedures for obtaining the pressed juice powder. This company is able to offer a highly effective and standardized nutritional supplement.

"I assure you that Carnivora® can be safely ingested and at low concentrations will produce the immune system supportive response noted by researchers and immune system monitors. Such research has been ongoing since the time I first observed how the Venus' flytrap caught and digested small insects coming within its outreach," states Dr. Keller. "In Dr. Morton Walker's next chapter (Chapter 5), I describe how I made my beginning acquaintanceship with the dining habits of Venus' flytrap in a flower shop."

The Fully Revealed Natural Components
of Carnivora®

The optimal oral intake of Carnivora® is one 125-microgram capsule taken three times daily for prevention of immune-compromising illnesses. In the event there is a life-threatening disease present already, Dr. Keller recommends ingesting up to six capsules daily. The safety of Carnivora® has been well substantiated through subacute (90-day) oral toxicity studies, negative mutagenicity, and genotoxicity test results. All of this substantiation has been carried forward by certified state laboratories in Germany. Carnivora® contains no pyrogens, endotoxins, or cytotoxins. It is one of the safest naturally derived therapeutic products ever used for the treatment of cancer. Here, revealed for the first time, is the full formulation of natural components present in Venus' flytrap juice.

The immune-supporting nutrient substances present in the phytopharmacon that Dr. Helmut Keller has named Carnivora® include the following:

- Droserone
- Hydroplumbagin-4-O-beta-glucopyranoside (listed here for the first time in the world medical literature)
- Diomuscinon
- Diomuscipulon
- Flavon glycosides: quercetin and myricetin
- Gallic acid derivates
- Arginine
- Aspargine acid
- L-threonine
- L-glutamic acid
- Glycine
- L-alanine
- L-cysteine
- L-histidine
- Proteases
- Lipopolysaccharides (paramune inducer)
- Phytohormones

When taken by injection or by mouth, the ingredients in Carnivora® bring about certain physiological effects for the human body:

- Carnivora® supports macrophage production and activity, including the formation of lymphocytes and the phagocytosis of granulocytes.
- Carnivora® supports the immune-stimulating effects of the chemical series naphthoquinones, which resemble those of photobol esters, known inducers of granulocytes.
- In immune-monitoring studies conducted by the biochemical laboratory Zytognost GmbH, in Munich, Germany, researchers reported that "the effect of Venus' flytrap pressed juice could be characterized as immunomodulatory. Its immune modulating effect is demonstrated mainly by a decrease of the white blood suppressor cells and an increase of the white blood helper cells, thus leading to the marked elevation in a debilitated cancer patient's all-important helper (CD4)/suppressor (CD8) ratio."

Venus' Flytrap, Venus's Flytrap, Venus-Flytrap

The correct spelling of *Dionaea muscipula* possesses three forms in common English usage. They are *Venus' flytrap, Venus's flytrap,* and *Venus-flytrap.* Any of these spellings is correct. Common usage has caused the carnivorous plant to be incorrectly spelled *Venus Flytrap.* Do *not* use this incorrect spelling!

Spreading from the base of Venus' flytrap are leaves three to six inches long, each of which broadens into a pair of kidney-shaped lobes that normally lie like a partially open book. These lobes act together like a steel trap when the prey, walking across the plant leaf, touches the base of the trigger hairs, causing the two lobes to snap shut. This is the most dramatic of all carnivorous plants.

In contrast to another carnivorous plant, the sundew, whose tentacles are tipped with a sticky exudate on which flying insects alight, the Venus' flytrap spreads out a rose-tinted, smooth carpet for crawling insects. Secretions inside the margin of the leaf act as a lure. The leaf has six slender hairs, spaced so as to form a triangle on each lobe. When a crawler touches two of these hairs (or one hair twice, since a double stimulus is necessary), the trap springs shut. Wind buffeting, raindrops, or sand particles do not activate the mechanism.

Venus' flytrap screens its prey by not immediately pressing too tightly. Tiny insects can escape through the spaces between the long, stiff bristles at the outer margins of the lobes. These bristles, which fold over loosely like the interlaced fingers of two clasped hands, form prison bars just for prey large enough to constitute a worthwhile meal. After a few minutes' time, the lobes of the leaf slowly press more and more tightly together, killing soft-bodied insects. Digestion is usually completed in five to ten days, whereupon the leaf opens wide again, ready for the next victim.[2]

Venus' flytrap bears white flowers in clusters on a stalk up to twelve inches long. Although it enjoys worldwide fame for the characteristic carnivorous behavior, this plant is native only to one small area, a strip of predominantly swampy ground covering perhaps as little as 700 square miles in the vicinity of Wilmington, North Carolina.

The Immunomodulating Components of Carnivora®

Developed as an effective treatment of malignant diseases and other impaired human immune states, Carnivora® is a standardized phytonutrient derived from *Dionaea muscipula*. The main immunomodulating component of the plant's juice is the phytochemical plumbagin with its hydrolysis product (molecularly split by water), hydroplumbagin-4-O-beta-glucopyranoside. These two substances are naphthoquinones, which appear as golden yellow, crystalline compounds that decompose at between 145°C and 147°C. They are soluble in benzene and ether and are related to the chemical substance 5,6-benzoquinoline.[3]

Together plumbagin and hydroplumbagin provide a variety of pharmacological properties, including antitumor, antibacterial, antiviral, and antiprotozoal activity. Additionally, the two components enhance actions of other immunomodulators, cardiotonics, hypolipidemics, and antibiotics. As an adjunctive agent or as solo treatment in oncological therapy, the Carnivora® phytochemicals optimize cellular defense by improving the pathologically deviated immune parameters.[4]

As cancer treatment, the therapeutic effect especially of plumbagin in Carnivora® is enhanced even more when another known anticancer compound is added to the treatment program as an adjunct. (Please see page 77 for a list of therapeutically adjunctive substances.)

In addition to pharmaceutically effective phytochemicals, mixtures of amino acids present in the pressed and refined Venus' flytrap juice include glycine, L-aspartate, L-threonine, L-glutamine, L-alanine, L-arginine, L-cysteine, L-serine, and L-histidine. Other less biologically active naphthoquinones in the fresh juice of *Dionaea muscipula* are droserone and 3-chloroplumbagin.[5,6]

Three institutional biochemists, one each from the University of Munich, the Hungarian Academy of Sciences, and the Pharmaceutical Research Institute of Hungary, who investigated plumbagin analogues in Venus' flytrap wrote: "The empirical application of *Dionaea muscipula* for cancer therapy is corroborated by data obtained in a detailed immunological investigation of all the major naphthoquinones, isolated from the plant. Only the substances plumbagin and hydroplumbagin-glucoside but not droserone and 3-chloroplumbagin show stimulating activities. Our observation that the enhancing effects could be triggered with unusually small doses of the active pure compounds correlates with the low concentrations of the same compounds present in the *Dionaea* extract [Carnivora®]. Our results support the notion that the antitumoral effect of the drug is due to immunoinduction."[7]

According to a report by Rumen Nikolov, M.D., Ph.D., D.Sc., professor and Pharmacological Department chief of the Chemical Pharmaceutical Research Institute, Ltd., in Sofia, Bulgaria, "The main pharmacological actions of plumbagin are that it shows broad spectrum antimicrobial activity against gram-positive and gram-negative microorganisms, influenza viruses, and pathogenic fungi. It offers antiparasitic activity against nematodes and malaria. Further, plumbagin in Carnivora® takes antiprotozoan action against *Leishmania braziliensis*, the cause of cutaneous leishmaniasis.

"More than that," continues Professor Nikolov, "in laboratory experiments I've witnessed antitumour activity for plumbagin in Carnivora® against rat fibrosarcoma and mouse leukemia. It has anti-anaphylactic action and a positive inotropic effect with cardiotonic action plus an hypolipidaemic and anti-atherosclerotic effect in rabbits. This substance enhances the activity of antibiotics by preventing the development of antibiotic-resistant cells. A negative for plumbagin is that it shows an antifertility effect by inhibiting ovulation and fertile egg implantation. Moreover, plumbagin is abortifacient."[8] Thus, according to Professor Nikolov, a pregnant woman should not take Carnivora®.

Indications and Toxicity of Carnivora®

There are standard human pathology indications for the administration of Carnivora®, and they include:

- Adult malignant tumors of all types
- Pain relief for cancer
- Blood dyscrasias such as leukemia
- Ulcerative colitis
- Crohn's disease
- Primary chronic polyarthritis
- Neurodermatitis

- Multiple sclerosis
- Immune deficiency diseases
- Acquired immunodeficiency syndrome (AIDS)

During the course of treatment with Carnivora®, the cancer patient usually experiences pain relief from cancer pathology. The relief commences within two to three weeks of therapy administration and continues as long as this potent phytopharmacon is taken.

Except for the potential of vein collapse from long-term intravenous injections of Carnivora®, there are almost no side effects from its use. The product is not mutagenic with no genotoxicity. And a study for acute toxicity among Sprague-Dawley rats indicates a mean LD_{50} ranging from 1,500 mg to 1,750 mg/kg of body weight.

Author's note: LD_{50} is the calculated dose of a toxic compound that causes death in 50 percent of a group of experimental animals to which it is administered. In pharmacology, the LD_{50} demarcation is used as a measure of the toxicity of drugs.[9]

Additional Lifestyle Practices for an Anticancer Program

Dr. Helmut G. Keller states: "The patient's helper/suppressor cell ratio is a mirror which reflects the power of self-defense in the control of cancer. This ratio is a key diagnostic figure. For treating malignant tumors, one must know that most immune-modulating compounds not only stimulate helper T-cells and natural killer cells, but they also excite the suppressor T-cells and suppressor macrophages. Immune modulators block cytotoxic lymphocytes and macrophages by releasing prostaglandins. It is therefore advisable to apply simultaneously prostaglandin-synthesis blocking substances such as indomethacin, piroxicam, buserelin, and silymarin."

Adjunctive Therapeutic Substances Employed with Carnivora®

The following is an alphabetical list of 105 remedial substances known to aid and support cancer patients. Oncologist Helmut Keller, M.D., employs one or more of them therapeutically for his patients as adjunctive measures to accompany Carnivora® treatment. These unconventional substances usually work synergistically with the pressed juice of Venus' flytrap to cause solid tumor shrinkage. They may also be effective by themselves or adjunctively with each other without the presence of Carnivora®. Most of them produce few adverse side effects (except synthetically produced drugs such as Amphotericin B®), and almost none of them are cytotoxic.

Remedial Substance	For Cancer and Other Diseases
ALJ® herbs: fenugreek, fennel, mullein, boneset, horseradish	Lung, bronchial, and brain metastases, viruses, digestive tract illnesses, anticonvulsive therapy
Amphotericin B® antifungal compound	All relevant fungal infections
Anningzochin® colony-forming *Mycobacterium chelonai*	Immunological enhancement
Anti-CD$_{44}$-IgG antibodies against CD$_{44}$	Glioma
Antineoplastons® per Dr. Stanislaw Burzynski's peptides and amino acids	Reprogramming of defective cells, destruction of invading agents or cells

APSI tumor vaccine for specific activation of immunity against remaining tumor tissue per Professor Tallberg	All malignancies
Aredia® pamidronate	Bone metastases
Aromatase inhibitors lower serum estradiol concentrations	Breast cancer
ASI tumor vaccine from patient's excised tumor tissue	Hypernephroma, ovarian cancer
Autologous immune therapy patient's blood enriched with antibodies, interferons, and interleukins	All solid cancers
Beres CSEPP Plus® 17 patented compounds (German)	All malignancies
Bio-Stim® glycoprotein klebsiella	Immune system building
BCG (Bacille-Calmette-Guerin)® tuberculosis vaccine	Bladder cancer, malignant melanoma
Caboran	All cancers for general tissue repair
Campto®	Colon cancer

Camu-camu from myrtle family, 100 g contains 2,000 mg vitamin C; doubles the glutathione level	Detoxification
Car-T-Cell®	Angiogenesis for spreading tumors
CSE blocker simvastatin and lovastatin for decrease of total cholesterol and LDL cholesterol	Neuroblastoma, CML, AML, ALL, CLL
Curcuma xanthorrhiza volatile oil	Antitumoral
DCA (body survival formula) desoxycholic acid produced from intestinal symbiotic bacterials	All cancers, immune boosting
DHEA dehydroepiandrosterone	Radiation and brain, breast, colon, lung, skin, lymphatic, gastric, prostate, bladder, and ovarian cancers; immune boosting
Essiac herbs: burdock root, sheep sorrel, turkey rhubarb root, slippery elm bark	Breast, prostate, colon, and pancreatic cancers
Enatone, Enatone/Gyn® leuprorelin acetate	Breast and prostate cancers
Ethanol (percutaneous injection of alcohol)	Liver cancer

Factor AF$_2$®   All cancers
biologic response modifier

Fetal liver   Prevention of cancer and
                                       micrometastases

Fish oil (EPA)   Immune system enhancement
eicosapentaenoic acid

Flaxseed/linseed oil   Bone and colon cancer,
linoleic acid   cancerobes (somatides per
                                       Gaston Naessens and
                                       Dr. Gunther Enderlein)

Foods phytochemicals,   All cancers, immune system
   antioxidants, enzymes: boosts
   tomatoes (vitamin C and
   lycopene), black and green teas
   (polyphenol), oranges and lemons
   (limoxin and glucarase), grapes
   (ellagen acid), onions (flavonoids),
   broccoli and cabbage (indoles),
   chili peppers (capsaicin), garlic
   (allicin), soybeans (see soy
   products below)

Gelum®   Activates metabolism, normal-
potassium, diferrum III triphos-   izes blood pH, vitalizes liver,
   phate, dipotassium ferrum III,   reduces ammonia, improves
   citrate complex   oxygenation

Germanium   T-cells, B-cells, NK cells, and
cells' mineral oxygen carrier   red blood normalization

Glucuronic acid blocks   Prevents metastases
   beta-glucuronidase enzyme

Glutathione (G-SH)
  mini-protein molecule

Antioxidant, inhibits carcino-
  genesis in the liver, nose, and
  throat

Goldstake® contains 22 minerals,
  including 20 mcg selenium

Prostate, breast, and other
  cancers for immune system
  boosting

H$_{15}$ (boswella plant acid resin)

Brain cancer

Heather root treatment
Calluna vulgaris

Leukemia, breast, cervical, and
  skin cancers

HER$_2$ monoclonal antibody

Breast cancer

Hoxey formula herbs: red
  clover blossoms, chapparal,
  licorice root, poke root, peach
  root, Oregon grape root, stillinga,
  cascara sagrada bark, sarsaparilla,
  prickly ash bark, burdock root,
  buckthorn bark, Norwegian kelp

Supportive in all malignancies

Hyaluronidase
hyaluronic acid enzyme

Softens cell membranes

Hydrazine sulfate
deprives tumor growth energy

Neuroblastoma, recurrent
  desmoid, Hodgkin's disease,
  lung cancer, and fibrosarcoma

Hyperimmune sera
gammaglobulin fraction from
  immune globulin IgG

Antigen for B-lymphocytes

Hyperthermia (heat therapy)

Most cancers

Immunotoxin   Blood-borne tumors
plant or bacterial origin lectin
   (ricin, saporin, abrin, gelonin,
   pseudomonas exotoxin)

Indomethacin (NSAID)   Inhibits prostaglandins, reduces
antirheumatoid agent   inflammation

IFR (interference current   All cancers
   regulation therapy) middle-
   frequency interference
   electric current

Jomol® fractions of rhodochrous   All cancers

Dr. Koch's treatment   "Survival factor" in neoplastic
carbonyl groups activated by   and viral diseases
   conjugation with double bonds
   of ethylenic linkages: quinones

Krallendorn®   Immune system plus bone, pan-
radix uncaria tomentosa alkaloid   creas, cervical, brain, bron-
                                      chial, lung, testes, prostate,
                                      and Hodgkin's cancers

Kreatin body's own compound   Energy
   arginine, methionine, and
   glycine

Lithium mineral   Radiation-caused leukopenia

Luffa extract from small Indian Amalgam and sinuses
   pumpkin   detoxification

Maitake® *Grifola frondosa*   Immune system
   Japanese therapeutic mushroom

Marimastat metalloproteinases blocking enzymes

Colorectal, ovarian, prostate, and pancreatic cancers

Miltex® miltefosin

Skin metastases in breast tissue

Melatonin neurohormone regulator

Anabolic process, regeneration of tissues, hormones, and enzymes

ML-1 lectin® mistletoe

Phagocytosis enhancer in all cancers

MVE-2 pyan copolymers

Immune system

Nemesis antidisease extract therapy by Dr. Sam Chachoua: viruses, bacteria, fungi, parasites isolated from cancer patient's serum and prepared as a vaccine

All cancers (see Chapter 10)

Neuraminidase receptor-destroying enzymes

Increases adhesion

Neunhoeffer's (Prof.) anticancer program activates xanthinoxidase and eliminates malignant cells' hydroxylamin metabolism

All cancers

Ney-Tumorin® animal organ lysates

Abdominal, lung, and bronchial malignancies

NO (nitric oxide)

Inhibits metabolic pathways to block growth

OK-432 *Microorganismus picibanil*

Immune system

Omega 3 and 6 fatty acids	Immune system
Ostac 520® clodrone acid	Bone metastases
Ozone O$_3$	Immune system by gamma interferon, interleukins, TNF, enzyme stimulation
P-30 *Rana pipiens* extract	Pancreatic and lung cancers
Padma 28 Tibetan herbs	Immune system boost by interferon production
Panorex® monoclonal 17 A-1 antibodies	Colon cancer
Parasite-killing program per Dr. Hulda Clark: black walnut tincture, wormwood, cloves	Kills cancer by intestinal fluke destruction
Percutaneous galvanotherapy per Dr. Rudolf Pekar, Austria	Skin tumors and breast cancer
Photodynamic therapy (PDT) photo sensibilation by photofrin II dye infusion which enriches tumor—then destroyed by laser light	Stomach, esophageal, anal, and vaginal cancers
PKS protein-bound polysaccharide *Coroilus versicolor*, a mushroom	Immune system
Pods $H_2S_2O_8$+H_2O_2+ethanol 96% peroxy-di-sulfuric acid	All cancers, especially prostate cancer

Polyerga® contains glycoproteins	All cancers by reducing fermentation
Q_{10} (coenzyme Q_{10}) ubiquinone	Breast cancer
Regeneresen® per Professor Dyckerhoff	Bone marrow repair
Ribozymes ribonucleic acids and hammerhead + tetrahymena enzymes	Colon cancer by gene neutralization
Ru-486® French abortion pill to block progresterone	Brain, prostate, and breast cancers and meningiomas
Shark cartilage	Antiangiogenesis for tumors
Selenium	Immune system boosting by binding toxic metals
Somatostatin antigrowth hormone	All abdominal and chest cancers
Soy products genistein and HEMF (4-hydroxy-2-ethyl-5-methyl-3(2H)-furanone)	Breast, stomach, and ovarian cancers
Spenglersan® *Mycobacterium bovis and Streptococcus pyogenes* colloids	Sarcomas
Suramin®	All cancers, especially trypanosomiasis
Taheebo hot holly tree bark tea	Leukemias, sarcomas

Thalidomide angiogenesis blocker	Kaposi's sarcoma plus breast and prostate cancers
Tamoxifen antiestrogenic	Breast cancer and malignant melanoma
Teboran mixture of aromates	Kaposi's syndrome and HIV-related conditions
Telomerase inhibitor enzyme DNA stabilizer	All cancers
Thymus calf thymus gland extract	All cancers by T-cell production
Ukrain® *Chelidonium majus*	All abdominal cancers
Urea	Breast and virus-induced cancers
Vincristin® Madagascar periwinkle	All cancers but especially breast, bronchial, neuroblastoma, malignant melanoma, sarcoma, plus Hodgkin's and non-Hodgkin's lymphoma
Vitamin E/beta carotene	Immune system plus lung, intestinal, and breast cancer
Vitamin B$_6$	Increase natural killer cells
Vitamin B$_{15}$ amygdalin (Laetrile)	Tissue oxygenation
Vitamin C	Detoxifies nitrosamines

Vitamin D	Bone and breast cancers, multiple myeloma, and bone pain
VBP 250 oleum carophylli, oleum thymi, menthol, oleum menthae pip., sunflower oil per Dr. Dieter Kaempgen	Kaposi's sarcoma and all virus-induced tumors
714X®nitramino-camper, NaCl, and ethanol per Gaston Naessens	All cancers by stopping somatides
Yucca tea yucca extract	Immune system and detoxification
Zinc mineral	Immune system
Zytocines IL-1, IL-2, IL-6, TNF, and alpha, beta, gamma interferon	Colon, kidney, ovarian, cancers plus myeloma, malignant melanoma, hairy cell leukemia, and micrometastases

Note: The above listing has been compiled by medical journalist Morton Walker, D.P.M., from information furnished by oncologist Helmut Keller, M.D.

Continues Dr. Keller, "Most cancer patients suffer from a severe disturbance in the area of the hypophysis, adrenal glands, and gonads. These endocrine conditions usually result in a distinct lack of corticotropin from uncontrolled tumor growth," Dr. Keller warns. "Such a problem should be balanced for the patient by substituting adrenocorticotropic hormone (ACTH) and/or dehydroepiandrosterone (DHEA).

"Also mandatory are changes for an improved lifestyle, including a well-balanced diet of fish or meat (never baked or fried or microwaved) that contains high amounts of protein," this German oncologist says. "The patient should ingest essential nutrients like beta carotene, vitamins E, C, and B_6 plus minerals such as selenium, lithium, zinc, and calcium, and lots of water. A daily detoxification procedure such as the Gerson Therapy must be followed too.

"Irrespective of the kind of cancer with which the patient must deal, he or she should live according to the rules of BLEST, my acronym for balanced nutrition (including detoxification and intestinal regeneration), love and laughter (approaching daily living with a positive spirit), exercise, sports, and temperance in all things," concludes Dr. Keller.

Resources

To receive more complete information about the natural and nontoxic alternative cancer therapies provided at the clinic offshore from the United States newly established by Dr. Helmut G. Keller, M.D., telephone toll free within the United States at (866) 836-8735 (866 VENUS FLY) or call from outside the U.S.A. at 001-(727) 781-0162.

Or, e-mail Dr. Keller at his commercial e-mail address: carnivora2000@yahoo.com.

Or, you may reach Dr. Keller for personal medical information at another e-mail address: doc h keller@yahoo.com.

Although it is best to communicate with him by e-mail, the home base for Helmut Keller, M.D., is Nikolaus-Feulner Strasse 22, D-96365 Nordhalben, Germany; telephone 011-49-9267-1702; fax 011-49-9267-1708.

The processed and purified Carnivora® pressed juice in the form of oral drops is approved for dispensing to patients and doctors by the German Health Authority (Germany's food and drug administration) known as *B farm* (previously called *Bun-*

desgesundheitamt or BGA). Carnivora® in its intravenous, intramuscular, and subcutaneous injectable forms are available by prescription directly from oncologist Helmut Keller, M.D. For prescription assistance, contact Dr. Keller at his personal e-mail address: doc h keller@yahoo.com.

Carnivora® may be acquired for cancer prevention, maintenance, and/or treatment as self-administered capsules and/or extract in the form of liquid drops by purchase from the manufacturer/distributor. To order capsules or liquid extract, contact Richard Ostrow, the owner, president, and chief executive officer (CEO) of Carnivora Research, Inc.; use the same telephone numbers as previously indicated: to the United States from overseas telephone 001-(727) 781-0162 or in the U.S.A. telephone toll free (866) 836-8735 (866 VENUS FLY).

The Carnivora® injectable solution awaits approval from *B farm* but may be available to some patients under the German FDA or the USFDA rules when Dr. Keller acts as the prescribing physician. Because of variables in legal regulations, sometimes the purified juice of Venus' flytrap can be obtained by other licensed physicians directly from Dr. Helmut Keller. Telephone to the manufacturer/distributor or to the physician/discoverer to learn why, how much, when to use and the answers to other questions about Carnivora®.

5

Other Effects of Carnivora®

Twenty-nine years ago, while driving from Boston to Maine to spend vacation time with his family, Helmut G. Keller, M.D., came across the Venus' flytrap plant. He had just completed a one-year medical internship at the Schlossberg Cancer Hospital in Oberstaufen, Germany, an institution linked to the Medical University of Munich. During this training engagement as an oncologist, Dr. Helmut Keller had tried to heal cancer patients by the application of cytotoxic therapies. His efforts usually ended in failure. "I had become totally disappointed with the horribly poisonous side effects of chemotherapy and was disillusioned with the oncology specialty I was electing to make my life's work. The question occupying my mind was, 'Should I continue as an oncologist?'

"On the ride to Maine I stopped at a flower shop to bring a gift of beauty for Elga, my loving wife. There I saw a number of the Venus' flytrap plants off in a corner of the flower shop and observed how they were catching and digesting bugs," Dr. Keller states. "The appetites of these plants for anything that crawled their way were voracious. I was fascinated with their feeding actions and remained in that flower shop watching for at least an hour.

"Afterward, I meditated on what I had seen and pondered about the Venus' flytrap's ability to assimilate and gain nutrition from insect (animal) protein," says Dr. Keller. "Perhaps, I wondered, they could do the same thing with human pathogenics and other such germs. Maybe the Venus' flytrap could provide enzymes to also 'digest' various primitive cells such as cancerous tumor cells.

"To stay alive, this herbal carnivore must be able to eliminate the 'simple' genetic codes of living animal protein that a Venus' flytrap ordinarily eats. My instinct told me that here was a possible treatment for overcoming malignant growths in humans," Dr. Keller concludes. "For me, it became worthwhile to invest study, money, and time in such a research project. I became determined to do that. Little did I understand then that applying the therapeutics of juice from the Venus' flytrap would become my life's work."

During the period when his evolving idea about Venus' flytrap enzyme juice was taking hold, Dr. Keller had already accepted a laboratory technician's position in a pathology research laboratory connected to Boston University. His full-time occupation was to administer different types of toxic drug treatments to formerly healthy laboratory animals—rats, mice, guinea pigs, hamsters, and dogs—which he had put into a state of ill health by inserting human cancerous growths into their tissues.

Utilizing his access to laboratory techniques, Dr. Keller set about investigating the digestive juices which allow the Venus' flytrap plant to sustain itself exclusively on flies, worms, mosquitoes, and other forms of living animal protein. One of his laboratory techniques included the colonizing of cancerous cells in vitro (in the test tube or petri dish) and then destroying them by their exposure to the enzymatic actions of Venus' flytrap juice.

Another laboratory technique Dr. Keller used involved the incorporation of cancer colonies into the cheek pouches of Syrian hamsters. Thus, he colonized cancerous cells in vivo (in living animals). Then, by extracting the Venus' flytrap juice from thriving plants, he proceeded to cure the cancer in the furry rodents.

The experience with his cancer treatment for hamsters held this inquisitive German-born physician in a state of joy, and he decided that he would remain in oncology. This positive mindset lasted a number of months for him until the FDA refused Dr. Keller's request to allow him to conduct a stage II clinical trial with Venus' flytrap juice on people who were victimized by cancer. He had unlimited access to cancerous patients coming to Boston's several municipal hospitals for free treatment. Under the informed consent doctrine, they were quite agreeable to participate in a clinical trial that might eliminate their cancers, but the FDA would not allow such experimental treatment to be administered.

Subsequently, Dr. Helmut G. Keller left his job at the pathology laboratory and returned to Germany with Elga and their children. There he established an experimental cancer treatment clinic in Bad Steben, a health resort town ("cure town" or "bath town" [Bad means "bath"]) devoted to offering tourists hot baths arising from the area's natural underground springs. In Bad Steben, Dr. Keller's Chronic Disease Control and Treatment Center specialized in administering immunostimulation, immunomodulation, and holistic medicine to cancer patients. Additionally he perfected the experimental applications of Venus' flytrap juice. Using his then newly formed manufacturing company, Carnivora-Forschungs GmbH located in his hometown of Nordhalben, he processed the Venus' flytrap juice in purified form, patented the process, and registered the purified Venus' flytrap enzymatic end product under the new trade name Carnivora®. (For more about Dr. Heller, see page 103.)

Immune Enhancements in the Human Body

It has taken him nearly three decades of laboratory analyses, clinical investigation, and the treatment of about 15,000 cancer patients, but now Dr. Helmut Keller knows how the purified plant juice does its work against human malignant tissue. He also has acquired a keen understanding of the human immune system. While long since having moved from Bad Steben to various other locations, in the interval Dr. Keller has made himself into an oncological immunologist with Carnivora® as the foundation for his effective immune enhancement therapy.

Few people know that each healthy Homo sapiens (human being) is equipped with an immune system cell count totaling more than 10^{12} of immune-competent cells (i.e., 10 trillion cells). If taken from the body and gathered all in one place, the immune system's disease-fighting cells would weigh approximately 1.5 kilograms (3.3 pounds) and are the main components of that invisible organ referred to as the immune system. This invisible organ may be considered an object of beauty. The immunity cells consist of a cocktail of macrophages which include millions of white blood cells (T-lymphocytes and B-lymphocytes). Such T-cells plus B-cells make up the blood's natural killer cells and plasma cells. Individual cells of the immune system are linked to each other through constant chemical feedback from within the body in response to harmful intruding microorganisms, foreign proteins, toxic metals, and other substances.

The human immune system also has a countermechanism that keeps its killer and scavenger cells from destroying normal healthy tissue and friendly organisms. The countermechanism consists of the blood's T-suppressor cells. T-suppressor cells possess the power to increase the human body's ability to kill incompatible organisms, and they work in conjunction with the T-helper cells to balance a person's immune system responses. The ratio between suppressor and helper cells determines how powerful the body's self-defense system is at any given time (in healthy people, the normal ratio is 1.2 ± 0.3).

Author's note: The T-helper/suppressor cell ratio acts as an indicator of the body's self-defense capacity and can be used to evaluate and monitor the health of an individual's immune system.

These are the regulating mechanisms that are inherited by all people as part of our human genetic makeup. However, the defense mechanisms can become diminished in persons with a history of physiological disorders. Even in healthy persons, the immune system can be lessened considerably by exposure to environmental pollutants, too much stress, and poor diet. To stay well, one must improve those conditions which diminish the health of one's immune system.

There is a solution available for offsetting illness-producing circumstances. Nature has provided us with numerous nutritional protective agents that support and enhance our immune systems. It's been learned that among the most advantageous nutritional supports is the phytonutrient Carnivora®. I have described it as having been derived from the juice of the Venus' flytrap plant.

Dr. Keller has proven that Carnivora® supplements mimic the body's own defense agents and support a stronger immune reaction. Those phytonutrient supplements developed by the American corporation Carnivora Research, Inc., maintain the carefully balanced immune system mechanisms. This enhances the immune system response in persons suffering from poor health, and maintains optimum immune response in otherwise healthy persons who are suffering from either internal or external stress.

How Venus' Flytrap Juice Acts on Animal Protein

"As I've stated earlier, in 1973, I discovered why Venus' flytrap juice is such an excellent dietary supplement for the human immune system," reiterates Helmut Keller, M.D. "Carnivora®

can be safely ingested and at low concentrations will produce the immune system supportive response noted by researchers and immune system monitors. The oral intake of Carnivora® is a single 125-microgram capsule taken two or three times daily for prevention."

For the presence of a life-threatening disease, Dr. Keller recommends taking two capsules three times per day before meals. "Carnivora's® safety has been substantiated by laboratories in Germany which conducted several subacute (90-day) oral toxicity studies." Dr. Keller continues. "They also acquired negative mutagenicity and genotoxicity test results, proving that the immune system enhancer I have discovered and then developed has no adverse effects. Carnivora® contains no toxic substances of any kind."

The immune-supporting nutrient substances in Carnivora® include:

- **Droserone:** 1,4-Naphthoquinone derivate
  Pharmacology: Spasmolytic, cough-blocking, antibiotic abilities
- **Hydroplumbagin:** Hydroplumbagin-4-O-beta-glucopyranoside
  Pharmacology: Immune stimulation and immune modulation
- **Formic acid:** Mono carbon acid
  Pharmacology: Antisepticum
- **Quercetin (flavonoid):** Quercetin-3-O-galactosid, -3-O-glucosid, - 3-O-rhamnosid, - 3-O-rutinosid
  Pharmacology: Antihemorrhagic, antisclerotic, antiphlogistic, antiedematous, dilatation of coronary arteries, strengthening of heart myofibrils (positive inotrop), spasmolytic, antihepatotoxic, choleretic, diuretic, estrogen effect, antioxidant, and chelating ability.

All of the different ingredients in Carnivora® have specific pathways in the human body, which contribute to improving and keeping up individual health in regard to immune system stimulation, supporting the circulatory system, and improving the heart's function.

- **Myricetin** (flavonoid): Myricetin-OH
  Pharmacology: Like the above quercetin
- **Gallic acid derivates:** Cholic acid, desoxycholic acid, and chenodesoxycholic acid
  Pharmacolgy: Emulgation of fat, facilitate the efficacy of lipases, immune stimulative, useful in degenerative and metabolic diseases.
- **Arginine:** (S)-2-amino-5-guanidinopentan acid
  Pharmacology: Essential in childhood, plays an important role in the uric acid cycle, liver protective, turns into the homologue of lysine, which is part of function in the mitochondria and participates in the production of creatine and putrescine, the pre-stage of spermine and spermidine, which stabilize the DNA structure in human spermatozoa
- **Aspargine acid:** Amino amber acid
  Pharmacology: Amino donator, so-called proteinogen amino acid
- **Threonine:** (2S,3R)-2-amino-3-hydroxybutan acid
  Pharmacology: Metabolizes to ketobutyrate and glycine, decreases cholesterol, protein element
- **Glutamine:** (S)-2-amino-glutaric acid
  Pharmacology: Donator of amino groups, detoxifying end product of ammonia metabolism, source of gamma amino-butyrate (neurotransmitter), acceptor molecule of ammonia detoxification
- **Alanine:** (S)-2-amino-proprionic acid
  Pharmacology: Key function is as glucogenic amino acid; it is essential to catalyze and block enzymes in the mode of action in penicillin
- **Cysteine:** (R9)-2-amino-3-mercaptopropionic acid
  Pharmacology: Causes acid urine, source of sulfate, high

concentration in the brain, essential for the fetus and premature children

- **Serine:** (S9)-2-amino-3-hydroxypropionic acid
  Pharmacology: Glycoproteins, component of immune globulins (antibodies)
- **Histidine:** (S)-2-amino-3-imidazol-4-yl-propanic acid
  Pharmacology: Metabolizes to histamine
- **Proteases:** Enzymes which split proteins and peptides; protein kinases, which block protein synthesis
- **Lipopolysaccharides:** Originate from the biosynthesis of polysaccharides, which bind lipids; retinol shows similar abilities
- **Phytohormones:** The source for gestagenes and estrones are sterines of tiny, unmeasurable amounts in the genuine pressed juice of *Dionaea muscipula*.

Carnivora® supports macrophage production and activity, including lymphocytes and the phagocytosis of granulocytes.

Investigation of Carnivora® supports the immune-stimulating effects of the naphthoquinones which resemble those of photobol esters, known inducers of granulocytes.

In immune-monitoring studies conducted by the biochemical company Zytognost GmbH in Munich, Germany, researchers reported that "the effect of Venus' flytrap pressed juice could be characterized as immunomodulatory, as demonstrated mainly by a decrease of the suppressor cells and increase of the helper cells, thus leading to an increase of the helper (CD_4)/suppressor (CD_8) ratio."

Up to 90 percent of all diseases are acquired by one or more factors from our environment. Only about 10 percent are still considered hereditary by medical science. The latter, hopefully, will improve in this century because of the advantage we already have by the identification of genetics. The main problem, therefore, is to decrease all the risk caused from the environment, in cutting down our exposure to electro-smog, avoiding chemicals and toxic or artificial compounds in our daily food, and much more. Daily physical exercise combined with positive mental attitude, intake of vitamins and minerals to assist in launching us to the point where we can expect to live as long as our genetic program determines our life expectancy (mankind is coded to live 120 years).

All of these precautions, however, don't solve the problems of different kinds of germs ("bugs") which are everywhere. They may trigger the mutations of our genes to a disastrous health condition, cause different kinds of infections which can be acute, but also be "hidden" until it becomes obvious by our deteriorating health.

The hazard of human pathogens such as fungi, viruses, bacteria, protozoa, and parasites are manifold. These germs can train and strengthen our immune system, which corresponds to the Chinese "yin." Alternately, an overload of the pathogens certainly contributes to the outbreak of the "yang" of which the end result becomes chronic diseases.

The individual expression of the different "bugs" is varied and multifold, depending on a patient's actual status, which includes the quality of his or her self-defense system. The immune system, this most important organ in one's body, has been disregarded in the past.

A wide range of different health problems is covered by a newly created food supplement, Carnivora® Immune Enhancer, which has been proven in the past decades of development to bring about the following effects:

- Antitumor activity by blocking protein kinases
- Increase of the self-defense power of our immune system, especially the T-cells and B-cells
- Broad-spectrum antimicrobial action against gram-positive and gram-negative microorganisms, especially for the influenza bacterium
- Action against RNA viruses, CMV, herpes, EBV, hepatitis

A, B, and C, and common colds; anti-leishmania, anti-malaria, anti-chlamydia, and anti-spirochete activity
- Enhancement of the action of antibiotics, due to their lack of effect on the antibiotic-resistant bacteria
- Cardiotonic action by increasing the pumping power of the myofibrils
- Hypolipidemic and antiarteriosclerotic effect
- Anticoagulant activity
- Antiallergenic and antianaphylactic action

The Carnivora® Immune Enhancer food supplement prevents and contributes to the successful treatment of all the above-related diseases and conditions. It improves daily life quality and life expectancy. No side effects are known. The Carnivora® dosage for prevention is one capsule three times per day before meals. The dosage to treat an actual chronic health problem is up to six capsules daily in divided doses of two before each meal.

A mode of action for Carnivora® was uncovered as recently as March 1999 by the KTB Tumor Research Institute, Inc., the laboratory division of the Institute for Molecular Medicine and Tumor Biology, in Freiburg, Germany. KTB discovered that the plant-derived product blocks nearly all the protein kinases (enzymes) of cancer cells, thus depriving a tumor of its ability to synthesize protein, which it needs to stay alive. Ordinarily protein kinases stimulate the development of cancer in three specific ways:

1. Tyrosinekinases, cyclin-dependent kinases of the cell cyclus, and protein kinase C, attached to the tumor's growth factor receptors, allow for unregulated and faster growth.

2. Other protein kinases regulate the programmed death of a cancer cell (apoptosis).

3. Protein kinases help to forward the signals for prolifera-

tion in the endothelial cells of blood vessel walls which feed the tumor (angiogenesis).

But Carnivora® inhibits all of these actions of the protein kinases and subsequently deprives the tumor of any ability to carry on its usual wild and excessive mitotic activity.

President Ronald Reagan Takes Carnivora®

Having therapies from around the world at his disposal and following the 1985 surgical excision of his colon's malignant polyps, U.S. president Ronald Reagan had sent to Nordhalben, Germany, for Carnivora® herbal extract to take as a preventive against potential colon cancer metastases. Thereafter, he drank thirty drops of the extract in a glass of purified water or herb tea four times a day. According to records kept by the extract's manufacturer, which was then Carnivora-Forschungs GmbH, the U.S. president continued to buy and swallow these drops until the onset of his Alzheimer's disease.

Even now it's suspected, but not confirmed, that Nancy Reagan uses Carnivora® for herself to avoid any recurrence of her breast cancer, and she continues to give it to her husband as well.

Nancy Reagan knows what she is doing. Although it may be taken orally merely for supplemental nutrition, Carnivora® drops and the newly developed soft-gel Carnivora® capsules have rather specific therapeutic applications. I have already listed some of them, but there are more.

Carnivora® blocks certain malignant tumor protein kinases and affords antimicrobial activity against most viruses, bacteria, and the trypanosomatid protozoa (leishmanias). It counteracts all kinds of human pathogenic microorganisms such as *Borrelia burgdorferi* (Lyme disease), *Helicobacter pylori* (gastric ulcers and gastric cancers), *Plasmodium falciparum* (malaria), staphylococcus, and numerous others.

Also Carnivora® offers cardiotonic action, hypolipidemic and antisclerotic effects, anticoagulant ability, and anaphylaxis inhibition. It has been used successfully for the treatment of chronic diseases including most forms of cancer, hepatitis A, B, and C, neurodermatitis, ulcerative colitis, Crohn's disease, multiple sclerosis, all types of herpes infections, primary chronic polyarthritis, and almost any immune deficiency state.

It is highly effective for the total elimination of the human immunovirus (HIV) in vivo from human blood and may be considered an effective treatment for AIDS.

As the "gold standard" for treating viral infections, Carnivora® has little competition. Its dried juice in a capsule attacks the actual viral organism, kills it, digests its toxins, and leaves behind dead viruses for debridement from the patient's bloodstream by phagocytosis. This Venus' flytrap extract works superbly to dissipate HIV. No other phytopharmacon or any other type of pharmaceutical considered useful in the treatment of AIDS does exactly what Carnivora® accomplishes—certainly not any of the frequently prescribed AIDS drugs such as Zidovudine® (AZT), Foscarnet®, Gancyclovir®, or Didanosine® (DDI). With no adverse side effects and at a fraction of the cost, the Carnivora® capsules seem more effective than the drugs for AIDS treatment.

Finally in the United States and around the world, therefore, we have access to Carnivora® Immune Enhancer capsules and liquid extract. This is a natural remedy from Germany, developed by cancer treatment pioneer Dr. Helmut G. Keller. It's the original dried, pressed juice of Venus' flytrap which promotes phagocytosis, blocks specific tumor protein kinases, contains antimitotic amino acids, enhances antibiotic activity, and generally provides a broad-spectrum antimicrobial action.

A Brief Profile of Dr. Helmut G. Keller

Born at 8:00 in the morning December 3, 1940, in the town of Erlangen, Germany, Helmut Keller was a "sunny, alert, and strong-willed baby," as his adoring mother recalls. During childhood he grew up in Erlangen and Amberg and passed his first years in grammar school uneventfully. The early deaths of Helmut's two siblings influenced his later decision to study medicine. He lost his sister, just two years of age, to a perforated appendix. Two years later, his small brother died from complications of a cystic kidney.

Helmut's parents decided that their remaining child deserved the best education available, and so they sent him to study at an exclusive private school on Lake Chiemsee in Bavaria. Part of their motivation was to move the boy into becoming more extroverted, for he was a somewhat withdrawn student who found his own company sufficient. Their plan worked, inasmuch as Helmut bloomed among the other children. He came out of himself, enjoyed any occasion to become enthusiastic with them over some activity, and laughed readily.

The young man developed a deep, honest, and abiding feeling for his fellow human beings, especially for the elderly. "As a youngster, I felt an extreme sympathy for older people, since I held this idea in my mind's eye," explains Dr. Keller. "I visualized them anticipating the death that was soon to come, and this vision made my heart ache."

In July 1963, he took his "Abitur" or school-leaving examination, which allowed him to study at the Friedrich-Alexander School of Medicine, University of Erlangen, from October 1963 to January 1969. More and more during those years of his medical training the young adult developed a deep concern for those patients that he observed in the throes of life-threatening situation. Trying to overcome an ailing patient's consuming chronic disease became his passion and full-time occupation.

After passing all of his examinations with the highest grades and going through internship in pediatrics, surgery, internal medicine, gynecology, and other specialty training, Helmut Keller received his medical doctorate in February 1970. His "approbation" or official sanctioning into the community of physicians worldwide occurred August 4, 1970. For a year thereafter, Dr. Keller took further training as a preceptor in the Department of Oncology at the Tumorklinik Oberstaufen.

From the Tumorklinik, he went on to the general practice of pediatrics, internal medicine, and surgery from October 1971 to March 1972. He was happy helping cancer patients, and he thought that there would be no barriers to his future. While working in the cancer hospital, he met his bride-to-be, Elga. But after a short time following his wedding, Elga's mother died at the age of fifty-three from cancer. It was then that Dr. Keller and his wife decided that they would move to her home in Boston, Massachusetts, where he took a laboratory research job offered at Boston University under the department chairman, Professor Fred Haendler. While working there he became fascinated with the animal protein digestive power of the Venus' flytrap and the concept of Carnivora® was born.

PART THREE

Additional German Cancer Therapies

6

Galvanotherapy

Not only nutrients and intravenous infusions are administered by European holistic/complementary/alternative CAM-type oncologists who use nontoxic and natural remedies against cancer; they also apply some highly sophisticated medical devices as well. Many of the devices include bioelectrical and/or electromagnetic components. Such machines have been reported by German-speaking doctors to provide patients with lifesaving cancer therapy that holds them in remission for indefinite periods.

Using the correct choice of voltage, amperage, and duration, the treating doctor can gradually attain every desired biological change in human tissue. From receiving mild electric current, the patient is not exposed to any toxic strain and at no moment is he or she in any danger. Galvanotherapy, the subject of this chapter, utilizes the natural tendency of electric current to deal with biological matter. The voltage usually does not exceed a value of 9.5 and is always less than 10 volts.

An electrical voltage administered to the skin at this lower value leads to the formation of fibrous connective tissue and the neutralization of malignancy. Fibroblasts and fibrocytes are the repairing components involved in fibrosis caused by the galvanic current. The bloodstream's macrophages phagocytize necrotic tissue produced during the course of therapy and takes it away as waste products.

Malignant tumors treated with electric current exhibit a change in their electrical charge. A portion of the cancer cells deteriorate and disappear almost immediately; sometimes they dissipate gradually in a relatively short time. Subsequently, the tissue becomes lighter as seen upon X-ray examination. Another part of the tumor's cells are inverted and reverted, that is, they first undergo differentiation, then form fibroblasts, and these repair cells integrate the area to bring it back under the natural control of the patient's organ, tissue, or body part undergoing galvanic treatment.

Galvanotherapy may be considered practically specific for the elimination of cancerous lesions, and nearly all of the time it exhibits a high rate of cancer removal success.

Galvanotherapy for the Elimination of Cancerous Lesions

By means of diligent applications of a biological electrical circuit to an anatomical area invaded by cancer, German, Austrian, Dutch, Italian, French, and other European holistic physicians are able to destroy solid malignant tumors. This bioelectric procedure, designated by the European oncologists who use it as *galvanotherapy* (GT), is generally unavailable in North America (except in Tijuana, Mexico). Canadians and Americans are denied GT because the treatment has not won approval from the continent's two major food and drug administrations (the Canadian Health Protection Branch and the USFDA). As a result of such official nonapproval, almost all North American health insurance companies refuse to pay for it even when GT eliminates tumors and saves lives. However, this method of galvanotherapy does permanently get rid of malignant growths far more effectively than any conventional mainstream cancer treatments currently administered. (See the cancer remission statistics coming out of China at the end of this chapter.) For example, GT works better than surgical excision because no residual cancer cells are able to remain after the completion of its application.

Describing the treatment with as little medical/electrical/technical language as possible, this brief chapter will provide the consumer with information on galvanotherapy as a means of eliminating cancerous lesions.

How Galvanotherapy Is Administered to a Patient

Galvanotherapy, a term originally used by its inventor, Rudolf Pekar, M.D., of Bad Ischl, Austria, has been broadly adapted by numbers of enthusiastic German-speaking physicians who apply the treatment. Dr. Pekar has now changed his mind about the term, however. He prefers another, more descriptive designation for his therapeutic method, *percutaneous bio-electrotherapy* or PBE. He calls it percutaneous bio-electrotherapy because the treatment works by means of an electrical field established with the help of electrodes clipped to needles inserted within the skin under local anesthesia in the region of a malignant tumor such as malignant melanoma.

In PBE, charged ionic particles move back and forth through the electrical field producing a kind of "melting" effect inside cancer cells. The result is that solid tumors tend to implode into themselves and the dead cancerous cellular tissue that is left behind becomes reabsorbed into the body's fluids as a waste product. The waste tissue then becomes eliminated over time during the individual's usual course of metabolic detoxification.

Using the reactions of weak electric currents on biological substances, cancer therapists are administering galvanotherapy as a physical technique of unproblematic, often painless reduction of tumor tissue. GT is applied as outpatient therapy. As already described, direct current (DC) of just a few milliamps is transferred into the malignant tumor, which hampers the growth of cutaneous (skin) cancer cells. Even in combination with conventional methods of cancer therapy, GP is transparent, safe, amazingly efficient, beneficial, and reproducible. This is a technique that is untraumatic to the body's organs. It does not require any hospitalization. And the treatment has a low price tag when compared to surgical intervention.

History of Pekar's Percutaneous Bio-Electrotherapy Invention

Dr. Rudolf Pekar, born March 29, 1912, studied at the Vienna School of Medicine. Shortly after the end of World War II, he started his private medical practice in Bad Ischl, Austria, in 1946. He first began to treat tumors with galvanic applications in 1969 and compiled a description of his clinical experiences for publication in 1988. It was in that first monograph that he first called the treatment of his invention *galvanotherapy*. The name has stuck despite his formally renaming the treatment *percutaneous bio-electrotherapy*.

Dr. Rudolf Pekar self-published another, fuller disclosure of his elimination work against cancerous tumors using GT or PBE in a second monograph during the latter part of 1997. It is an elegant little book translated from German to English.

In April and May of 1999 when I began investigating German cancer therapies from my base of operations at Klinik Winnerhof in Bad Wiessee, Bavaria, Germany, Dr. Pekar contacted me through my friend and cancer consultant Helmut Keller, M.D., and asked that I, as a medical journalist who specializes in writing on complementary and alternative medicine (CAM), provide broader exposure for his cancer treatment. The doctor wanted to allow more patients access to the benefits of his therapy's efficacy for cancer. He believed that galvanotherapy or bio-electrotherapy was too little known outside of German-speaking medical circles, and he was correct.

Today, at age ninety-one, the inventor of galvanotherapy wants to leave behind a legacy of healing. Consequently, he has provided me with written permission to quote freely from his 1997 monograph, and I have done so. Here you are offered my interpretation of what has been published in the monograph *Percutaneous Bio-Electrotherapy of Cancerous Tumours* by the treatment's inventor, Dr. Rudolf Pekar.[1]

The Physiological Mechanism of Anticancer Galvanotherapy

With great success, the Pekar treatment has already been administered to an estimated 65,000 patients throughout Europe and a few other parts of the world. The bio-electrotherapy (BET) used for galvanotherapy has advantages over surgical intervention. BET does not provoke metastasis. It does not stress the cancer patient's total being (his or her physical body, psyche, emotions, and inner spirit). Frequently its nonanesthetized application hurts in the form of a stinging electric current. But this stinging or burning sensation may be controlled effectively by local injections of lidocaine, xylocaine, or another dental-type anesthetic at the administration site of GT.

Negatively charged particles called *anions* migrate to the positively charged pole, an *anode*, in the electrochemical cell. Positively charged particles called *cations* migrate to the negatively charged pole, a *cathode*. Between the poles, a charge separation or *dissociation* occurs. This dissociation damages malignant tissue in the following manner: Extremely acidic tissue plus chlorine is generated at the anode; conversely, a markedly alkaline environment plus hydrogen is generated at the cathode. According to their charge, small and large ionic particles, such as those in proteins, separate inside of the electrical field. The cancer cells caught between this electrochemical reaction completely depolarize, so that they become permeable and accepting of various substances poisonous to them. Meantime, therapeutic agents are being administered intravenously to the patient. Thus, the tumor tissue at the treated site can no longer maintain its specific equilibrium, and it destabilizes.

Types of Tumors Responding to Galvanotherapy

Particular tumor types respond well to galvanotherapy. Under the ministrations of Dr. Rudolf Pekar and his oncological colleagues, this form of electrotherapy is successful for eliminating the following malignant conditions:

- Breast cancers
- Mouth and throat cancers
- Esophageal and stomach cancers
- Lung cancers
- Vaginal cancers
- Melanomas and basal cell carcinomas
- Skin metastases
- Lymph node metastases
- Liver metastases
- Mycosis fungoides
- Rectal cancer and anal cancer

From the use of GT for malignant tumor removal, the advantages are many. Such benefits consist of the following:

- The organ involved is preserved with no problematic scarring.

- The electrical needles are applied under local anesthesia without risks.
- None of the side effects which may be connected with general anesthesia are present.
- No damage occurs to healthy tissue.
- As a result of lysed tumor components being presented to the immune system for removal, an additional immune stimulation takes place.

From receiving galvanotherapy, certain types of cancer patients benefit greatly. Such malignancy patient types include:

- Those with small primary tumors of less than 5 cm in diameter
- Those with solitary metastases, especially in the skin and lymph nodes
- Those with recurrences in the region of an operation such as a mastectomy scar
- Those who possess external but inoperable tumors

The Introduction of Bio-Electrotherapy into China

In addition to Rudolf Pekar, M.D., who administers bio-electrotherapy from his office clinic at the Onkologische Schwerpunktpraxis in Bad Ischl, Austria, five other oncologists have participated with him in gathering statistics solely related to their galvanotherapy applications for cancer. The five physicians are Swen Alfas, M.D., chairman of the Academy for Applied Knowledge International in Frederiksberg, Denmark; Friedrich Douwes, M.D., medical director of the Klinik St. Georg in Bad Aibling, Germany; Giuseppe Gasso, M.D., oncologist in chief at the Centro Catanese di Onkologia in Catania, Italy; Xin Yu-Ling, M.D., the cancer clinic director at the China-Japan Friendship Hospital in Beijing, China; and Helmut Keller, M.D., former medical director of Klinik Winnerhof, Bad Wiessee, Bavaria, Germany. These outstanding oncologists who utilize CAM techniques for reversing cancer are prime exponents of galvanotherapy.

From his own experience with cancer treatment, Dr. Rudolf Pekar advises us regarding the average success rate of galvanotherapy when administered for any and all types of cancer. He says that a 73 percent rate of remission for not less than three years is the figure he can state definitely that bio-electrotherapy achieves. He does qualify his statement with the words: "It should be noted, though, that in my practice, I have only been able to treat mild and moderate tumors."

In 1988, Nobel laureate Professor Bjorn E. W. Nordenstrom, M.D., Ph.D., of Stockholm, Sweden, introduced electrochemotherapy with galvanotherapy as a primary component to Chinese healers. By 1993, this treatment was already being performed in 818 hospitals throughout China. The Chinese medical community had picked up on galvanotherapy with great vigor in the same way they had readily adapted the porcine splenic extract, Polyerga®, for their ailing cancer patients. Bio-electrotherapy impressed them with its quick-acting electromagnetic fields of healing.

The 200-year-old model of biological matter introduced by Dalton in 1808 is still widely used in the science of medicine within China. This model is based on a highly simplified assumption that matter consists ultimately of indivisible discrete atomic particles. The attraction of atoms to each other leads to a chemical reaction. Binding forces between the atoms are visualized along abstract lines as in the meridians of acupuncture.

Besides the chemical reactions between matter, an additional, more profound countereffect has been observed since Dalton introduced his theory. Matter, particularly biological matter, radiates electromagnetic fields at all times. And Dr. Rudolf Pekar, even as a young physician, realized this fact. He states in his book: "Every biological process is also an electric process. Health and sickness are related to the bio-electric currents in our body."

This conclusion of Pekar's is a new paradigm for understanding biological substance. The therapeutic application of that knowledge and the introduction of electric current into the tumor with needle-electrodes are epoch-making ventures. The influence of electricity on cancer cells is profound. Those Chinese physicians aware of Dr. Pekar's concept have recognized its importance far in advance of physicians practicing conventional allopathic medicine in North America.

Healing Statistics for Galvanotherapy Reported out of China

As a result of the First International Conference of Bio-Electrotherapy (BET) for Cancer held in Beijing, China, in 1992, a statistical breakdown of the treatment's administration showed the results of applying galvanotherapy for all types of tumors in 2,500 cases. Every one of the cases had been presented to the conference attendees by Chinese medical scientists (see Table 6-1). Their statistics indicated that for a wide variety of malignant tumors more than 35 percent of the cancer patients experienced complete remissions (CR). And almost 43 percent showed partial remissions (PR). Over 15 percent could report no change (NC); and less than 7 percent exhibited progressive disease (PD). Table 6-1 offers a summary of the Chinese medical experience with the use of galvanotherapy (bio-electrotherapy) for malignant tumors.

Statistics for the patients' case histories tell the whole story of treatment efficacy. The participating Chinese doctors' experience is undeniable, and their therapeutic responses from cancer patients are extraordinary. There should be absolutely no reason for continuing to deny patients residing in North America access to receiving galvanotherapy for malignancy elimination.

Table 6-1
Cancer Reduction Efficiency of Bio-Electrotherapy as Experienced by the Administering Oncologists in China

Cancer type	Patient Load Number (#)	CR #	CR %	PR #	PR %	NC #	NC %	PD #	PD %	CR + PR #	CR + PR %
Lung cancer	593	168	28.3	298	50.3	76	12.8	51	8.6	466	78.6
Liver cancer	389	98	25.2	196	50.4	74	19.0	20	5.1	294	74.7
Skin cancer	366	244	65.8	95	26.0	20	5.5	10	2.7	336	91.8
Breast cancer	288	78	27.1	82	28.5	59	20.5	9	3.1	160	55.6
Metastatic lymphoma	190	49	25.8	89	46.8	31	16.3	21	11.1	138	72.6
Rhabdomyo-sarcoma	113	29	25.7	56	49.6	19	16.8	9	8.0	85	75.2
Malignant melanoma	95	56	58.9	34	35.8	4	4.2	1	1.1	90	94.7
Facial tumor	72	28	38.9	29	40.3	11	15.3	4	5.6	57	79.2
Metastases in breast and abdominal wall	66	17	25.8	25	37.9	15	22.7	9	13.6	42	63.6
Thyroid cancer	57	20	35.1	24	42.1	9	15.8	4	7.0	44	77.2
Oral cancer	53	11	20.8	34	64.2	5	9.4	3	5.7	45	84.9
Total	2,516	885	35.2	1,080	42.9	379	15.1	172	6.8	1,969	78.3

Key: CR is complete remission, PR is partial remission; NC is no change; PD is partial deterioration.

The Three-Year Remission Rate for BET or GT

At the Second International Conference of Bio-Electrotherapy for Cancer held in Stockholm, Sweden, in 1993, the Chinese oncological participants reported that their galvanotherapy administrations to 4,000 cancer patients resulted in an accumulation of complete remissions and partial remissions (CR + PR) exceeding 80 percent. This remission rate is better than any other reported therapy for malignancies. It far outshines chemotherapy and radiation therapy as delivered in the United States. The American Cancer Society (ACS) considers chemotherapy to be beneficial at only a 5 percent response rate. How would the ACS classify galvanotherapy? The answer is that the ACS labels galvanotherapy as "experimental" or "investigational" or "unconventional." The Chinese have given GT legitimacy because the three-year survival rate for Chinese cancer patients receiving galvanotherapy lies well above 70 percent.

Similar or even better results than those clinical studies published in China were achieved with galvanotherapy for all types of cancers by Professor Giuseppe Gasso, M.D., of Catania, Italy. Worldwide, the estimated average percentage of three-year remissions arising from the application of galvanotherapy is about 72 percent for most types of tumors and cancer stagings. From the written hand of the Austrian inventor and expert on bio-electrotherapy, Rudolf Pekar, M.D., the best average three-year remission rate he has experienced is 73 percent. (Unlike those in the United States, European oncologists consider that "near-cure" has been achieved for a cancer patient in the presence of a three-year remission.)

Resources

To be educated more fully about applying the science and techniques of galvanotherapy/bio-electrotherapy, contact Rudolf Pekar, M.D., president (*Praesident*) of the International Association (*der Int. Ges.*) for Electromedicine (*fuer Elektromedizin e. V.*) at his cancer specialty practice (*Onkologische Schwerpunktpraxis*), Frauengasse 4 (Villa Gisela), zip code A-4820 Bad Ischl, Austria; telephone 011-43-6132-22511 or alternatively 011-43-6132-23244; fax 011-43-6132-23244-3. He often speaks English through an interpreter, Hubert Laaber; telephone to Herr Laaber at 011-43-6132-2456-8.

The elegant monograph written by Dr. Rudolf Pekar, *Percutaneous Bio-Electrotherapy of Cancerous Tumours*, may be acquired from its editor, Gerhard Grois at Wilhelm Maudrich KG, medical publishers, A-1096 Wien, Spitalgasse 21a, Vienna, Austria; telephone 011-43-1408-5891; fax 011-43-1408-5080; or by ordering it directly over the Internet at the publisher's website: www.maudrich.com. The price is $54.00 per copy.

7

Whole Body Hyperthermia

In 1883, an American general surgeon, William B. Coley, M.D., operating out of Memorial Hospital in New York City, picked up on the 1868 published medical report of a little-known family physician named Peter Busch, M.D. Dr. Busch had written that he successfully treated sarcoma of the face in a forty-three-year-old woman who underwent what was described then as a "spontaneous" cancer cure. It had happened directly after she overcame the skin infection erysipelas.[1]

Part of the established symptom complex for this erysipelas illness and its bacterial cause, Group A, beta-hemolytic streptococcal infection, is a full body fever. It's not unusual for the fever to rise as high as 105 degrees Fahrenheit (105°F). In fact, Dr. Busch reported that his patient did attain fevers ranging from 40 degrees Celsius (40°C) to 41°C (the equivalent of 104°F to 105.8°F).[2]

Recognizing that an elevated temperature is the body's way of naturally coping with invading microbes, Dr. Coley decided to experiment with laboratory animals that had been given various forms of cancer. It took him almost twenty years to develop and apply clinically what we know today as Coley's toxins. In 1906, Dr. Coley published a complete description of his work with bacterial toxins derived from *Streptococcus pyrogenus* and

Bacterium prodigiosum (also known as *Serratia marcescens*), which he injected into human patients suffering from advanced cancers. Using the Coley toxins, he induced fevers in his cancer patients ranging from 38°C (100.4°F) to 42°C (107.6°F).

Although this researcher described impressive results during three decades of treatments, in particular against osteosarcoma and soft tissue sarcoma, Dr. Coley's method did not become popular until recently (starting about 1980) due to the inhomogeneity of his bacterial batches. Also there were certain severe microbial complications for his patients.[3]

Still, Dr. Coley did establish the hypothetical value of full body fever for the treatment of particular cancers. Therefore, Robert C. Atkins, M.D., medical director of the Atkins Center in New York City, supposedly predicts his anticancer program on Coley's toxins combined with an alkaloid such as ukrain or the plant *Sanguinaria canadensis* in the family of bloodroot. The alkaloids raise the body temperature as high as 107°F. The combination of Coley's toxins and the alkaloid is administered ten or twelve times, each time at a little higher dosage, with most patients reportedly showing a positive response.

The hypothesis of heat therapy against cancer had been further entrenched in 1957 when three statistically minded oncologists reviewed 450 cases of so-called spontaneous remissions of histologically proven malignancies. They found that at least 150 remissions from the total were associated with acute infections and physiological responses from the patients' naturally elevated body temperatures. The oncologists' published report in *Cancer Research* was significant, but it remained unheralded. In the United States and Canada, consequently, heating the body as a cancer therapy continued to be ignored for perhaps another twenty-three years by most of the North American oncological community.[4]

Not so in other parts of the world such as Germany, France, Italy, the Netherlands, and Austria. Whole body hyperthermia (WBH) was especially drawn to the attention of certain enlightened German physicians who use CAM. Experimentation with raising the body's inner core as a viable anticancer treatment began in earnest in Germany. Even in that country, however, the allopathic oncological community was opposed to any therapeutic technique which varied from the established surgical, chemical, and/or radiation therapies. The allopaths, as they do routinely for anything deviating from what is usual and customary in medicine, put up immense resistance to WBH. The result is that WBH has been held back for decades, and the specific victims of such political infighting which involves the practice of medicine have been the suffering cancer patients themselves.

Heating the Body as a Cancer Therapy

At the Cleveland Clinic in the United States, another progressive general surgeon world-renowned for his work with breast cancer, George Crile, Jr., M.D., held no fear of butting heads with his allopathic medical colleages. Aware that the outcomes of most malignancies had been only minimally improved by the existing conventional cytotoxic treatments, Dr. Crile took an interest in tissue heating as a therapy against cancers, especially sarcoma. He also recorded an interest in that 1957 statistical evaluation showing human cancer remissions from fever therapy and subsequently performed his own laboratory investigations. Dr. Crile published two journal articles which discussed his in vivo animal studies with heating malignant cells and tissues as a potential cancer treatment.

In the Crile experiments, the cancer line S180 sarcoma, implanted in the left foot of a mouse, was subjected to the same local elevated temperature as the normal opposite (contralateral) foot of the animal. Dr. Crile showed that while the malignant tumor could be destroyed by exposure to 44°C (111.2°F) for 30 minutes, 200 minutes at the same temperature were required to damage the healthy foot. By modifying the time and temperature levels, Dr. Crile concluded:

- Destructive effects of heat on malignant tissue begin at 42°C (107.6°F), and for each degree above this temperature the time required to produce the same biological effect is halved.
- For any given time of exposure the temperature required to cause destruction of normal tissue is 3°C (5.4°F) higher than that needed for destruction of a malignant tumor.[5,6]

Other investigators later presented well-documented data on animal tumor models which responded to elevated temperatures.[7] Some medical researchers combined heat with ionizing radiation and cytotoxic agents to achieve a tumor-killing effect in laboratory animals. Both of these forms of cancer cell destruction are enhanced by adjunctive application of local, interstitial, regional, or whole body hyperthermia (see definitions below).[8,9,10]

Of major significance, in fact, is the evidence that hyperthermia potentiates the antineoplastic effects of various therapeutic modalities—even the toxic ones like radiotherapy, chemotherapy, and immunotherapy. Such evidence had led to important clinical applications in the treatment of human cancer. In 1934 and 1935, for instance, demonstrations were held in which malignant tumors were heated during or after radiation therapy. Because of heating the involved tissues, X-ray dosages required to induce cancer regressions were sharply reduced.[11,12] Moreover, there was a radiosensitizing effect of heat shown to occur on murine tumors. While a dose of 5,000 cGy was required to cure 50 percent of tumors, one hour of tissue exposure to heat up to 43°C (109.4°F) reduced the required roentgenological dosage by a factor of three.[13]

Radiobiological studies indicate that hyperthermia and ionizing radiation are effective against different components of cancer cell population and thereby can exert synergistic cell-killing action when applied together. Several biologically important factors are responsible for this beneficial effect.[14]

WBH Machines Sold Around the World

The construction pioneer of hyperthermia machines sold around the world was South Carolinian Harry Leveen, M.D., who died December 28, 1996. Dr. Leveen began building hyperthermia devices for delivery in the United States over thirty years ago. However, his few American-made hyperthermia units for local or regional body application by means of radio frequency never won approval for United States distribution from the U.S. Food and Drug Administration (FDA). They were banned in this country, and Dr. Leveen was forced to ship them for storage at the University of Bangor, Wales, in the United Kingdom. These units, now labeled "British hyperthermia machines," were sold by Dr. Leveen's sales agents to the various countries of Europe and to Japan.

While it is hardly utilized in America, hyperthermia as an anticancer modality is well established in nearly every Western industrialized nation of Europe. Indeed, the application of heat for the treatment of human malignancies is presently under intensive study in many medical centers throughout the world, as stated, in particular by oncologists practicing in Germany, Austria, France, Holland, Italy, and currently Mexico.

During a telephone interview I conducted with Vera de Winter, Ph.D., administrator of the Veramedica Institute of Munich, Dr. de Winter said: "The St. Georg Klinik of Bad Aibling, Germany, has more than seven years of clinical experience with the use of systemic whole body hyperthermia and has treated over two thousand patients. From application of such elevated heat, the average remission rate for patients with advanced stages of cancer is 80 percent. There is no other treatment modality known with such a high remission rate.

"Those patients who exhibit advanced tumors of the liver, lung, pancreas, bone, colon, stomach, kidneys, prostate, peritoneum, mediastinum, large intestine, and other sites where cancer has already broken through the intestinal wall can benefit from the combination of low-dose chemotherapy and systemic whole body hyperthermia," Dr. de Winter said. "Whole body hyperthermia has shown itself to be safe and well tolerated, even by debilitated patients. Such systemic hyperthermia has provided successful results for advanced tumors, and it has an impact on distant metastases as well.

"Twelve years ago I became acquainted with Dr. Harry Leveen. At that time I traveled to the University of Bangor in Wales looking for the last of his hyperthermia machines which might still be available. Dr. Leveen helped me to find a Leveen local hyperthermia device to bring to Germany, and that's when I founded the Veramed Kliniks and Hospital of Brannenberg, Germany for special cancer treatments," continued Dr. de Winter. "I engaged Dr. Friedrich Douwes, a very advanced physician, to be the chief of medicine of my hospital. We used a Leveen local hyperthermia device to treat cancer patients for the first time ever in Germany. In 1992, Dr. Douwes and I left the Veramed Kliniks and Hospital. Then Dr. Douwes established his own place, with all the freedom in medicine a true biological physician requires, and he has continuously progressed in the techniques of adminstering hyperthermia using various modalities to kill the different malignant tumors."

Using local hyperthermia in the form of a catheter with a heating antenna at its end that he invented, Dr. Douwes reported to me that he is experiencing a 90 percent success rate in reversing prostate cancer for his patients. The antenna, passed through the penile urethra, also works well as the means of shrinking prostate enlargement that's responsible for benign prostatic hyperplasia (BPH).

Knowing that I was recording his remarks for publication, Murray "Buz" Susser, M.D., of Santa Monica, California, former president of the American College for Advancement in Medicine (see the ACAM membership listing in Appendix B), told me that he had traveled to Munich to receive BPH treatment from Dr. Douwes. A normal prostate is about 25 grams. And as a result of his local hyperthermia, Dr. Susser's gland diminished from a measurable 45 grams to just 30 grams in size. He has experienced a reduction of nocturia from three times nightly to the normal number of urinations—none or just one.

The Techniques of Administering Hyperthermia

In October 1997, the Twentieth Annual Congress on Hyperthermia was held in Baden-Baden, Germany, as part of Medicine Week. Just about every Western country, except the United States and Canada, was represented by a medical speaker giving a paper on hyperthermia. There was so much information to present that the hyperthermia part of Medicine Week lasted for three days. On May 28, 1998, a follow-up hyperthermia conference was held in Venice, Italy.

Hyperthermia, the use of heat in the treatment of human cancer, is delivered to the patient by three main approaches in clinical practice:

1. Whole body hyperthermia (WBH), in which systemic temperature is raised to at least 42°C (107.6°F)

2. Regional hyperthermia, in which the part of the body containing the malignancy is heated either by perfusion with heated fluids or by deep heat applications

3. Localized hyperthermia, in which the heat is focused di-interstitial hyperthermia, a subtreatment under the category of local hyperthermia, the heat is administered by an antenna at the end of a probe injected into the body of a cancerous tumor.

The artificial induction of heat for therapeutic purposes is most effective in the range of 42°C to 44°C (107.6°F to 111.2°F). Ideal is 108°F. Below this range little cellular damage occurs; above it, as was shown in animal experiments conducted by Dr. George Crile, Jr., the sensitivity of normal cells begins to approach that of malignant cells, and damage to normal tissue may result.[15,16] Additionally, Jozef Mendecki, Ph.D., and his colleagues at the Radiation Therapy Department of Montefiore Medical Center, Albert Einstein College of Medicine, located in the Bronx, New York, subjected a group of C3H mice to four sessions of heating at 42°C (107.6°F) delivered to a transplanted mammary carcinoma. Not using any accompanying toxic treatment, but just hyperthermia alone, was the Mendecki team's approach. In all treated mice the cancer regressed and disappeared; the mice remained well and survived for several months beyond the researchers' expectations. In the control, untreated mice, the cancers grew rapidly and all animals died within four weeks.[17]

Seven years after Dr. Mendecki's experiment, another pair of cancer investigators duplicated his result, but the tumor regressions of their laboratory animals were either partial or of short duration when hyperthermia was used alone.[18] Correct technique in applying hyperthermia is absolutely vital for the best therapeutic response.

I interviewed Dr. Jozef Mendecki, who is associate professor of radiation oncology at the Albert Einstein College of Medicine. Today he does his research in the Department of Urology at the affiliated Montefiore Medical Center. For many years while a member of the medical school's Department of Radiation Oncology, Dr. Mendecki treated patients with various forms of cancer using a combination of hyperthermia and radiation therapy. Presently his research concerns the development of a new approach using hyperthermia in the treatment of benign prostatic hyperplasia (BPH). He provided me with an immense amount of information for this chapter and other works of mine in progress.

Dr. Mendecki advised that when whole body hyperthermia (WBH), combined with ozone, is inserted extracorporeally (outside the body) into the patient's blood, infection with viral pathogens such as with the human immunodeficiency virus (HIV), may be eliminated. This combination, ozone and WBH, furnished by the extracorporeal method, becomes a viable treatment for the victims of acquired immunodeficiency syndrome (AIDS). Both ozone and WBH are antimicrobial. But neither mechanism is used extensively as treatment for AIDS. They simply are being overlooked.

Extracorporeal whole body hyperthermia and externally applied systemic whole body hyperthermia are delivered mainly for the elimination of most types of cancer. Also they can be combined effectively with low-dose chemotherapy and low-dose radiation therapy.

Extracorporeal Whole Body Hyperthermia

In Mexico City, heart surgeon Carlos Fink Serralde, M.D., who also treats cancer, described his method of administering extracorporeal WBH. Dr. Fink explains, "First we sedate the patient, and then we make a needle puncture for insertion of a catheter into the right femoral artery and on the opposite leg into the left femoral vein, both near the groin. A closed circuit is thus established. In between these two inserted catheter tubes we connect a heat exchanger for heating and cooling. Blood is used as the heat transfer medium to raise core body temperature.

"Next, we raise the heat exchanger's temperature to bring the body temperature to 42°C [107.6°F]. That's done by the patient's blood being heated extracorporeally. Meantime, we have placed thermometers in the patient's esophagus, rectum, and autotransfusing blood to observe that the body's temperature remains elevated near to 108°F," says Dr. Fink. "While blood can be heated extracorporeally as high as 48°C [118.4°F], a person's body temperature remaining at 108°F is perfect for cancer therapy. The circulating blood stays at that level for either one hour or one and a quarter hours, depending on the supervisor's judgment.

"The patient experiences his heated blood circulating at the rate of 400 cubic centimeters (cc) per minute. This is quite slow compared to the blood flow of four meters per minute during open heart surgery," states the cardiac surgeon. "For hyperthermia the attached machine is merely a heat exchanger; for open heart surgery, a heart-lung machine is pumping blood around the body. The speed of blood-pumping action needs to be much faster during heart surgery than for raising the body's temperature. After the heating time limit has elapsed, we cool down the blood to normal, remove the catheters, and send the patient for a followup with local radiation therapy, if it's required. In Mexico City, we never administer chemotherapy with hyperthermia and often use extracorporeal whole body hyperthermia by itself."

A patient's core temperature of 42°C is critical in extracorporeal WBH. Multiple temperature measurements of brain, bone, and a variety of other organ sites show uniform temperature levels equivalent to usual core determinations. For example, 42°C in the rectum will show 42°C in the bone marrow or in the brain. Temperatures below 42°C are often ineffective. Reaching 43°C (109.4°F) is more effective for killing cancer cells, but that elevated body temperature is likely to be more difficult for patients to tolerate. In fact, sustained temperatures above 43°C may cause liver damage or brain injury. Active liver disease or injury is a relative contraindication for WBH, although patients with hepatitis C have cleared their infections following WBH for cancer.

As indicated by Dr. Fink's prescribing sedatives prior to WBH, any injury to the central nervous system of patients is avoided by the use of those sedatives. Available to the patient may be intravenous anesthesia with benzodiazepines and inhaled oxygen. Although rare, cardiac problems are a possible adverse side effect of this type of extracorporeal heat therapy.

Externally Applied Whole Body Hyperthermia

In contrast to Dr. Fink's extracorporeal type of WBH, the Douwes method of systemic whole body hyperthermia (SWBH) may attain slightly lower core temperatures, ranging from 41°C (105.8°F) to 42°C (107.5°F). For elevating body temperature, Professor Friedrich R. Douwes, M.D., medical director of the St. Georg Klinik and Hospital in Bad Aibling, Germany, uses a high infrared light within an enclosed unit. As described by Dr. Vera de Winter, what follows is the procedure employed at the Veramedica Institute of Klinik St. Georg in Bad Aibling.

"Prior to SWBH, the patient is prepared for treatment by undergoing an extensive clinical examination and laboratory tests. During the treatment itself, the patient lies in a special fabric enclosure that looks like a rectangular-shaped tent. Intensive care monitoring is conducted," Dr. de Winter advises. "At the start of treatment, the patient is administered a cytokine combination injection of interferon, IL-2, and lipopolysaccharides. This combination stimulates the immune system and brings about a slight fever reaction; however, it's insufficient to produce heat damage in the tumor, so that an infusion of 20 percent glucose is given as well. This infusion raises the blood sugar level to above 300 mg percent [hyperglycemia].

"Together, the fever reaction and the hyperglycemia produced at the same time bring about a massive stimulating effect on the patient's immune system. The immune reaction leads to additional overacidification of the cancerous tissue," said Dr. de

Winter. "Then there's the targeted introduction of heat provided by an infra-red A light which furnishes infra-red A light radiation of 85 to 1,300 nm as a result of its special adjustable radiation reflector system. The radiation light spectrum is matched to the human skin and thus penetrates deeply into the body. The blood circulation ensures that there is a goodly supply of energy to the body core.

"The special radiation reflectors producing the infra-red A light lead to gradual heating in the capillary bed of the subcutaneous connective tissue. More heat is generated than can be given off, and this produces a slow, controlled rise in temperature to any level required between the normal body temperature of 37°C [98.6°F] and 42°C [107.6°F]. For the treatment of cancer, body temperature levels ranging from 40.5°C to 42.2°C are considered therapeutic. But extreme hyperthermia from 42°C upwards is only tenable under anesthesia by supervision of an anesthetist," Dr. de Winter concluded.

Hypotheses of How WBH Works
Against Cancer

Although he has actively engaged in studying all forms of hyperthermia for more than twenty-two years, Dr. Jozef Mendecki says, "The exact mechanism of cell inactivation by heat is not clear. We know that heat in the hyperthermic range inhibits the synthesis of vital macromolecules such as DNA, RNA, and proteins. Also it causes depression of multiple cellular enzymatic systems, possibly resulting in impairment of cell replication, and may explain why malignant, actively cycling cells are more readily damaged by heat than are normal cells."

Dr. Mendecki's statement is predicated on information uncovered in 1980 by a group of ten medical researchers working together.[19]

The effect of heat on organelles is thought to be mitochondrial damage, according to Dr. Mendecki, and this results in a reduction of oxidative processes with a depression of metabolism. In a tumor cell, such heat damage further decreases an already low pH. The acidity, in turn, stimulates lysosomal enzyme production. Since the heat additionally increases lysosomal membrane permeability, the enzymes are released into the cytoplasm. There is a massive outflow of enzymes from the cancer cell which leads to cell digestion.[20]

A growing malignancy can be viewed as a self-impoverishing organism; as it grows farther away from a well-vascularized periphery, its central portion becomes deprived of oxygen and nutrients. Thus, it becomes more acidic. Under these conditions, the tumor turns more heat sensitive. No doubt, all cells become more vulnerable to heat under conditions of low pH, poor oxygenation, and nutritional deprivation.[21]

Heat as a physical agent against cancer or microbial infection or for other types of nonmalignant disorders such as Stages I and II hypertension, systemic disorders of localized but widespread rheumatic forms like scleroderma, and for treatment-resistant neuralgia, requires but two parameters for its activity. They consist of time (duration) and temperature level (intensity). The minimum time required to produce irreversible cell damage at a given temperature has been designated the thermal death time (TDT).

In seeking the TDT, a hyperthermia therapist must be wary of bringing about an interesting aspect of resistant cell response. The therapist must know that just one nonlethal thermal treatment of mammalian cells (including cancer cells) can modify and even drastically reduce their subsequent response to heat. This transient resistance is called *thermotolerance*, and has been found to last from forty-eight to seventy-two hours. It's believed that the unique molecular mechanism arises from certain "heat shock proteins" synthesized during this nonlethal but conditioning period.[22]

When done correctly, hyperthermia enhances immunological reactions that contribute to a better cancer cure rate. As examples of excellent cancer healing, I cite rectal carcinoma and melanomas. There are fewer metastases in patients treated with external systemic and/or extracorporeal whole body hyperthermia for melanomas when amputation is delayed by four weeks after hyperthermia.[23] Patients undergoing electrocautery for rectal carcinoma had fewer metastases than patients treated with surgery alone.[24]

Heated tumors act as an antigenic source. Pathological slides of malignancies subjected to hyperthermia show marked infiltration of lymphocytes and macrophages in the vicinity of the target tissues. There is enhanced immunogenicity of at least some cancers by the heat therapy's ability to unmask cell surface antigens of the cancerous cells.[25]

Certainly this simple method of using hyperthermia—local, regional, or whole body—for exposing cancer cells to the human immune system's protective mechanisms is a viable way to accomplish the growth reversal of cancer.

A Case History from the St. Georg Klinik

"I'll present to you the situation of a very famous German actress and singer, who had suffered from ovarian cancer with metastases to the liver and the lungs," clinical oncologist Professor Friedrich R. Douwes, M.D., explains. As indicated previously, Dr. Douwes is medical director of the Veramedica Institute, an affiliate of the St. Georg Klinik and Hospital in Bad Aibling, Germany (near Munich). "My patient then was fifty-three years old and much admired for her acting on the stage, in films, and in soap operas during daytime television. She has gone public with her cancer experience and has described it on many talk shows broadcasted throughout the German-speaking world. You can tell her story to the world." *(Author's note: Since I did not receive the actress's personal permission to identify her, I've chosen not to reveal her name.)*

"The first manifestation of her ovarian cancer was in 1991 when my patient underwent cytotoxic drug treatment at Munich University. She relapsed for the first time in 1993 and again was administered chemotherapy. Next, a relapse occurred for her in June 1996, but she did not react positively to additional chemotherapy given then. Months of progressive illness followed," Dr. Douwes said.

During further discussion in the course of our interview, the oncologist told me about ovarian carcinoma. It most frequently manifests itself in the fifth decade of life, causing fluid pooling, swollen legs, and pain in the intestinal area and in the backs of the legs. There is abnormal vaginal bleeding, weight loss, and changes in urination and bowel movement patterns. Dr. Douwes' famous patient was approaching death. Then her friends, colleagues, and family prevailed upon the actress to take whole body hyperthermia treatment under his supervision. Dr. Douwes is internationally known for his nontoxic, biological therapies against cancer and cancer pain.

"Her admirers appealed to me to help this woman. They said, 'She is so much loved, so talented, and so famous. We want to have her alive. Please, can't you do something for her?' I saw her at the St. Georg Klinik for the first time in January 1997. When she arrived, the patient suffered from ascites. She was troubled by a liver infiltrated with cancer, and her left lung had shut down from the cancer's metastases. She had severe hoarseness of the voice, hardly able to speak both from shortness of breath and from paralysis of the vocal cords," explained Dr. Douwes. "Then she was treated here with whole body hyperthermia. My patient went into complete remission of her ovarian cancer. She has no more ascites and no liver infiltration. Her lung is completely open, vocal cords working well, and she is back on stage for several years now. Today she sings beautifully.

"Just before Christmas 1997, the actress visited me for a physical checkup, and I was able to report to her that all organs in her body are functioning properly and her laboratory readings are normal. The ovarian cancer, including its metastases, are gone," Dr. Douwes advises. "She told me, 'I'm back to work acting and singing, and I want to give you a present. I'm going to perform a one-woman musical for you, the clinic staff, and all the patients.' We have a spa here, you know, so the actress took over our auditorium building (known as the Kurhaus) for a two-hour show.

"Much media was in attendance—newspaper reporters, television crews, radio commentators, and other press people from all over Germany," Dr. Douwes describes. "I was interviewed on television and radio over and over. The press asked me, 'What did you do? It's a miracle!' But I replied that this is no miracle; it's just correct medical application of whole body hyperthermia. I have no doubt, as this type of heat treatment gets known, more and more patients will become healed of their cancers. The death sentence given by doctors to cancer patients that 'you have only so many days or weeks to live' will no longer exist."

Resources

To acquire more information about hyperthermia, especially the whole body type, contact the nonprofit foundation Survive Until a Cure, Inc. It's devoted to prolonging the extent and quality of life of terminal patients afflicted with AIDS and inoperable cancer. Survive Until a Cure, Inc., may be reached by telephoning (203) 227-LIFE, i.e., 227-5433, or e-mail: survive@sprynet.com.

You may also contact Friedrich Douwes, M.D., St. Georg Hospital, Hyperthermia Centre, Adalbert-Stifter Strasse 4, 83043 Bad Aibling, Germany; telephone internationally 011-49-8061-

498-0; fax Int. 011-49-8061-498-455; e-mail: info@klinik-st-georg.de; website: www.klinik-st-georg.de.

Or contact Vera de Winter, Ph.D., N.D., Veramedica Institute, Braunstrasse 7, 81545 Munich, Germany; telephone 011-49-8964-7692; fax 011-49-8964-2285-9; mobile telephone 011-49-17-1270-0797; e-mail: veramedica@aol.com.

8

Noni Therapy

From his Bay Eye Clinic in North Bend, Oregon, ophthalmologist John T. Flaxel, M.D., advises that he and his wife Joy are concerned about a longtime personal friend currently suffering from mammary carcinoma with metastases to the liver. Writing to the renowned oncologist Friedrich Douwes, M.D., at his Klinik St. Georg in Bad Aibling, Germany, Dr. Flaxel reports, "Our friend, Mary Anne L., a single parent with a teenage daughter, has had three recurrences of breast cancer over the past ten years. Recent additional chemotherapy was not helpful."

The interpretation that Dr. Douwes made of this patient's laboratory and clinical information which arrived from Dr. Flaxel is: "She obviously has extended breast cancer and is now in the stage of drug resistance." Persuaded by the ophthalmologist, Ms. L. made an effort toward her own recovery and did travel to Bad Aibling for treatment with whole body hyperthermia and other oncological remedies. Included among several nostrums administered by the German oncologist for effective adjunctive application has been phytochemical adaptogenic healing with noni therapy.

"The noni therapy I dispense to my patients is manufactured by American Nutriceuticals, Inc., located in Sarasota, Florida,"

Dr. Douwes stated during our Bad Aibling interviews on April 26, 2001. "I use this brand because I am convinced that this company makes excellent anticancer remedies. I have compared several noni products and observed their immune effects in my cancer patients. The many noni liquids available cannot compare to results achieved with the noni juice capsules. They work while the various liquids do not. I see that the capsules bring about beneficial immunomodulation for cancer patients, which is the sole reason I prefer to use noni juice capsules.

"My routine practice is to perform a series of blood tests before and after giving a cancer patient one of my immune-boosting remedies. I call this type of product testing for the patient an 'immune check.' It offers me an important indication as to whether taking the nutriceutical, phytochemical, vitamin, mineral, enzyme, or some other anticancer remedy is going to be advantageous for my patient," says Dr. Douwes. "I also do a lysis test of the patient's cancer cells using certain computer measurements, following the ingestion of an oral or injectable remedy. If the remedy is going to bring my patient improvement, the computer shows that existing malignant cells go into the lysis state. They seem to fall apart or explode. Noni is one of those natural and nontoxic substances that cause cancer cell lysis."

Two weeks prior to my visit with Dr. Friedrich Douwes, Dr. John Flaxel had mailed information to me about his cancer-ridden friend who currently lives in Paris. He wrote: "She has undergone basic care with detoxification and nutriceuticals [including the noni therapy], so that her liver metastases have gone away. The liver tumors' disappearance was indicated by an MRI [magnetic resonance imaging] as visualized by her French physicians.

Author's note: Mary Anne L.'s sister is a Parisian radiologist, and this relative's medical colleagues are monitoring treatment results for the patient.

"Our friend's tumor markers are now normal," Dr. Flaxel

continues. "Her neck mass has almost disappeared too, and blood tests show themselves to have returned to normal. This woman looks and feels the best that she has in years. I hear from the family that the patient's French doctors can't believe it [what they're observing]. I hold a recent medical report documenting her improvement, and it verifies her medical progress toward complete healing [from ingesting noni juice capsules]."

A week after mailing me this information, the ophthalmologist added in a telephone interview, "Our friend's swollen supraclavicular cancerous nodes have gone away; she has done amazingly well. As part of her cancer care, in addition to other things, her doctors have followed my recommendation and have put her on [a higher dosage] of noni. While previously she had been designated by [conventionally practicing] oncologists to have perhaps only five months to live, my friend's upward leap in improvement has been remarkable for those physicians who know her case. Noni is now part of a total program of treatment for this person," says Dr. John T. Flaxel. "And you can use this case history to illustrate some of the adaptogenic healing offered by noni therapy."

Daniel Dugi, M.D., Makes Noni a Routine Part of His Therapies

As an owner and staff member of the Physicians' Family Health Center in Cuero, a town in south-central Texas, Daniel Dugi, M.D., says: "I dispense noni juice capsules and other herbals extensively in my family practice, but noni is the most essential ingredient that I use for alternative health care. It has become a routine part of my therapies for almost everyone. I employ it for the treatment of hypertension, cancer, inflammatory arthritis, systemic lupus erythematosus, and most other connective tissue diseases. Without question noni capsules manufactured by American Nutriceuticals, Inc., are among the most efficacious of all the many immune-boosting products used by holistic medical practitioners. Noni therapy provides my patients with the most incredible healing effects.

"A good example is the fifty-six-year-old woman I will identify as Mrs. Gladys S. Gladys, whom I saw this morning, is the victim of both lymphoma and leukemia; I started her on noni therapy four weeks ago. Today, her swollen axillary lymph nodes which had been filled with malignant tissue are totally gone. Last week the oncologist who is taking care of Gladys telephoned me and asked, 'Dan, what have you recommended to be taken by Mrs. S. as a nutritional supplement? Her lymph nodes are just melting away.' Having observed this effect, the patient's oncologist is just amazed and wants to know more from me. In fact, this was the third recurrence for Gladys, and her doctors were running out of treatment options for her," Dr. Dugi says. "Previously, I had been offered no opportunity to dispense noni with its associated botanical products, Ecomer® and Badmaev 269™, to Gladys but now this combination is saving her life by increasing the immune system's response."

Author's note: All three nutritional supplements benefiting Dr. Dugi's patient, Ecomer® Shark Liver Oil Alkyglycerols, Badmaev 269™, Tibetan herbal ingredients, and encapsulated noni powder, are manufactured and sold by American Nutriceuticals, Inc. (please see the Resource section).

"*Morinda citrifolia* shows significant antitumor activity by means of a significant reaction from animal and human T-lymphocytes; it has a humoral response too, for I've seen immunoglobulins improve dramatically just by putting cancer patients on noni therapy. Thrombocytopenia corrects itself by elevation of the cancer patient's thrombocytes from 40,000 per ml of blood to 100,000 after just two months on noni," affirms Dr. Dugi. "The noni acts as an adaptogen to rebalance malfunctioning systems and bring them back to normal. Also it affords an energy boost—modulating the body's energy. Noni has definitely become an integral part of my treatment protocols for almost all patients.

"My father is a lung cancer survivor; I made the diagnosis when his tumor was only four millimeters in diameter, located in the lingular segment of his left lung. He had the area resected, and from taking noni for the past ten years my father has done exceedingly well," Dr. Dugi says.

"For me, too, noni has done a good job. Arthritic inflammation in the joints of both my hands along with movement limitations in my back disappeared after I took noni capsules for a mere three weeks. When I discontinued taking the noni for eight days, my inflammations returned swiftly, but upon returning to noni the inflammation went away within two weeks. So now I personally stay on the capsules all the time. Ingesting the manufactured capsules coming from American Nutriceuticals, Inc., is good preventive medicine," affirms family physician Dan Dugi, M.D.

Enlightment About the Plant That Provides Noni Therapy

Being apprised of patient progress against cancer, one may wonder as to what medical science tells us about the derivation and uses of noni. Has there been verified research performed on the substance—does the research tell us what it is and what it does? After I have waded through multilevel marketing hype about noni fruit and juice, the medical journalist report you are reading offers corroborative information about this innovative biologic. Here, there is no hype.

Growing best on soil composed of highly mineralized volcanic ash in the open coastal regions of China, India, Indonesia, the Philippines, Samoa, Tahiti, Hawaii, and other regions of the South Pacific, a small evergreen tree or bush or shrub classified as *Morinda citrifolia* is used broadly by native medicine men. This tree, thriving in Hawaii because of its volcanic soil, is classified as belonging to the botanical genus *Rubiaceae*. It has rigid, coarse branches that bear dark, oval, glossy leaves. Small white fragrant flowers bloom out of clusterlike pods that bear creamy-white colored fruit. The fruit is fleshy and gel-like when ripened, resembling a small breadfruit.

Ancient Healing Ways for the Fruit of Many Names

For more than two millennia traditionalist healers around the Pacific Rim have prized this evergreen. Centuries ago the native healers named it "noni" in Hawaii and defined its use by the extra names "painkiller tree" and "headache bush." Of all the world's regions that produce *Morinda citrifolia* for medicinal purposes, the Hawaiian noni is cited repeatedly by therapists as the most effectively healing. Its preventive and health-producing components consist of the plant's bark, stem, root, leaf, and especially the fruit.

As had been the practice for over two thousand years and is still done today, the traditionalists administer noni components for a wide variety of health problems, including sinusitis, arthritis, digestive disorders, colds, flu, headaches, microbial infections, menstrual problems, accidental injuries, pain, skin disorders, and a great deal more. Kahunas, those traditionalist healers or native doctors of the Hawaiian Islands, are the greatest exponents of noni, which they utilize as an adaptogen—a daily tonic—for its normalizing function, immune system support, anti-inflammatory characteristic, joint mobility restoration, analgesic effect, and other overall health benefits. In the United States and nearly all other Western industrialized nations, medical doctors, osteopaths, chiropractors, naturopaths, nutritional consultants, herbalists, and additional health professionals also recommend noni, but they dispense it usually in encapsulated powder form that is derived as an extract processed and dried from the noni fruit.

The noni tree produces this prized fruit, which grows up to 12 cm in diameter. Such fruit results from a coalescing of the inferior ovaries of many closely packed flowers. Despite noni fruit's foul taste and soapy smell when overly mature (too ripe), for centuries the plant's bark, stem, root, leaf, and fruit have been taken internally as a folk remedy for numerous degenerative diseases including diabetes, hypertension, cancer, and a great many additional health difficulties.[1,2]

Noni is considered by medical scientists, anthropologists, and health-care historians to be the most important plant brought to Hawaii by the first Polynesians.[3] When completely ripe, flesh of the noni fruit produces a very distinctive odor; when overripe, unfortunately, the rancid smell of fermentation is overpowering.

The manufacturer/distributor, American Nutriceuticals, Inc., refuses to extract noni powder for encapsulation from fermenting fruit. It picks fruit selectively and then immediately starts its proprietary process of juicing the whole noni fruit. Next, the juice product is freeze dried to -5°C (-20°F).

How Noni Powder Is Extracted for Encapsulation

The South Pacific plant *Morinda citrifolia* has had a vast amount of research performed on it to determine aspects of its therapeutics. Nutritional scientists recognize that the rich volcanic ash that overlies all of the Hawaiian Islands grows noni fruit offering the best healing effects. Specially processed fruit extract that is powdered and encapsulated provides the most benefit when administered for treatment of human pathology and for preventive medical purposes. In part, the method by which noni powder is extracted for encapsulation determines its efficacy.

Each plant possesses five, eight, or ten pods that hold three to five fruit in each pod clump. The fruit ripens at various stages. American Nutriceuticals workers selectively harvest the noni fruit in its golden color which offers the peak of enzymatic activity. Golden-colored noni far surpasses the therapeutic effectiveness of any other colored noni fruit. The golden yellow fruit is especially better than whitish-colored noni with its effacing membrane and beginning fermentation.

Noni fruit colors range from a deep forest green when the pod is new, hard, and rocklike. It then changes to a light green with still-hard fruit clusters. Upon noni's becoming golden yellow in color, the knowledgeable harvesters for American Nutriceuticals search it out and pick it. Their harvesting must be quick because the fruit's natural enzymatic action changes its skin from golden to translucent white, and this alteration occurs between twenty-four to forty-eight hours. At this later stage, the noni invariably becomes unpickable. Touching it allows a harvester's finger to go through the fruit's membrane (the outer wall). With any aging, noni becomes mushy and unusable (although some noni juicing companies accept such fruit for processing). Mushy noni indicates rotting fruit and should be rejected.

Besides selective harvesting, American Nutriceuticals, Inc., certifies that its encapsulated powdered product is free from herbicides, pesticides, irradiation, fumigation, and fruit fermentation according to standards set by the U.S. Food and Drug Administration (FDA). A traditional way of harvesting noni is to place the picked fruit on rattan mats to dry in the sun; a month later, it is processed for human consumption. Such an old-line technique of drying the fruit tends to allow too many undesirable bacteria (upwards of 2 million cultures per gram) to grow. For ridding the drying noni of so much bacterial growth, germicides in the form of deadly chemicals are employed or fumigants are sprayed on it or the noni is irradiated. No method of bacterial kill is healthful for human beings.

With regards to the American Nutriceuticals, Inc., processing of *Morinda citrifolia*, company officials can honestly say their product is free of germicides, fumigants, and irradiants. The FDA allows such claims, and that is significant for the health of consumers.

Another aspect of the company's unique production methods is that the whole fruit is used, including the seeds and skin, to provide all the nutrients that nature intended. Once the noni fruit is crushed for faster drying and lesser bacterial contamination, it is flash frozen to -5°C. Such flash freezing stops the denaturing process that hits any picked fruit. Like the aloe plant, noni also possesses an immense amount of polysaccharides which would denature if left unattended. After the flash freezing, noni is then freeze dried—an effective commercial method of extracting water from the fruit. Resulting from the manufacturing process is a 10 to 1 concentrate of whole fruit to whole noni juice powder.

What American Nutriceuticals, Inc., prepares and sells is noni juice in powdered form with the only substance removed being water. Thus, the end product will have never been heated to high temperatures, which could compromise the fruit's enzymes; no excipients or binders or flowing agents are ever added either. Capsules are the cleanest noni product available—it's 100 percent fruit and juice (never the leaves) of *Morinda citrifolia*. While not certified as organic, the American Nutriceuticals product has been grown under organic conditions.

Known Chemical Compounds in Noni

Publishing an important 1999 article in the *Journal of Agriculture, Food and Chemistry*, ten scientists discussed the chemical compounds in noni. These ten biochemists currently are staff members of three scholarly institutions: the Department of Food Science and the Center for Advanced Food Technology at Rutgers University, the Department of Food and Nutrition at Osaka City University, and the Pacific Biomedical Research Center at the University of Hawaii. In their article they described their isolation of two glycosides, asperulosidic acid and rutin, plus a trisaccharide fatty acid ester from the extracted n-butanol-soluble fraction of the fruits of *Morinda citrifolia*. These chemicals were shown to prolong the life span of mice implanted with Lewis lung carcinoma by stimulation of the animals' immune systems.[4]

Additional compounds from noni also exhibited antitumor activity. Damnacanthol and anthraquinone, both isolated from the chloroform extract of the roots of the noni plant, inhibited the malignancy's *ras* function and suppressed activated *ras*-expressing tumors. Extracts made from noni roots also possess some significant dose-dependent, central analgesics which affect mice.[5]

Noni seeds are used as a laxative; its leaves alleviate skin inflammation and pain; the roots lower blood pressure; the bark is an antimalarial remedy; the flowers treat eye inflammations; and the noni fruit is held in reverence for its ability to do a massive number of good things for mankind. Harvey Kaltsas, D.O.M., L.Ac., whose interview is reported in my next subsection, writes in *Alternative Medicine* magazine that "noni combats bacterial infections (as an antibacterial), clears the lungs and eliminates mucous conditions (as an anticatarrhal agent), heals inflammation (as an anti-inflammatory), softens and protects the skin (as an emollient), promotes and regulates menstruation (as an emmenagogue), lowers elevated blood pressure (as an antihypertensive), regulates the bowels (as a laxative), calms the nerves (as a calmative), and clears poisons from the body (as a detoxifier)."[6]

Several active ingredients are present in noni juice and the encapsulated dried powder created from this juice. The tree's putative active ingredient is proxeronine, an alkaloid which becomes converted in the living organism (in vivo) to xeronine.[7] Additional therapeutic agents present in noni are ricinoleic acid, found in the seeds,[8] morenone present in the roots,[9,10] and the anthraquinone glycosides with flavone glycosides from the flowers.[11] Finally, small quantities of the vital phytochemicals beta-sitosterol and ursolic acid are found in the small tree's leaves.[12,13]

Chemical constituents in noni may be categorized according to the parts of the evergreen tree from which each constituent derives. Not every part of the plant is used for therapeutic purposes. For completion of the reader's knowledge, however, all of the ingredients actually present in each noni plant are listed below accompanied by a notation as to their use:[14]

- In the fruit (used extensively). Working their therapeutic effects are caproic and caprylic acids; essential oils; B-D-glucopyranose penta-acetate 2; asperuloside tetra-acetate; glucose; and ascorbic acid. Also present is the alkaloid labeled proxeronine, the precursor to xeronine. Finally, there is damnacanthol, which inhibits viral growth and cellular mutations involved in cancer development.

- In the leaf (not used). Amino acids are present including alanine, arginine, aspartic acid, cysteine, cystine, glycine, glutamic acid, histidine, leucine, isoleucine, methionine, phenylalanine, proline, serine, threonine, tryptophan, tyrosine, and valine. Added to them are anthraquinones, glycosides, phenolic compounds, resins, beta-sitosterol, and ursolic acid.

- In the flower (not used). Present are the three natural chemicals having the formulas: acacetin 7-O-D (+)-glucophyranoside; plus 5,7,-dimethyl apigenin-4-O-8-D(+)-galactophyranoside; plus 6,8,-dimethoxy-3-methyl anthroquinone-1-O-8-rhamnosyl glucophyranoside.

- In the root and root bark (not used because the noni plant would be killed by their removal). Found as ingredients are the nutrients:

alizarin	sodium
chlorubin	morindine
chrysophanol	sterols
ferric iron	carbonate
morindadiol	soranjidol
rubiadin	magnesium
anthraquinones	glycosides
rubichloric acid	resins
phosphate	

Harvey Kaltsas, D.O.M., Recommends Noni for Immune Stimulation

Speaking with me from his office in Sarasota, Florida, doctor of oriental medicine Harvey Kaltsas, DOM (OMD), D.Ac., confirms: "I do a lot of nutritional consultation for cancer patients, and taking noni is my usual recommendation for such persons. Noni is highly beneficial for immune system stimulation, especially when it's employed synergistically with other herbals such as Ecomer® and Badmaev 269™. These three botanicals in combination from American Nutriceuticals respond well to my testing them with electroacupuncture diagnosis.

"Noni in particular stimulates the production and activity of white blood cells and seems to aid in the leukocytes' more effective targeting of cancer cells. For instance, I've seen a number of prostate cancer patients, a couple of lung cancer patients, a liver cancer patient, a peritoneal cancer patient, and a sarcoma patient all respond well to the ingestion of noni juice capsules produced by American Nutriceuticals, Inc. I believe that noni is one of the most essential botanicals to be used to bring about recovery from cancer," says Dr. Kaltsas. "A chemical in noni, scopalatine, is strongly suspected as the source of the fruit's immune system stimulation.

"Upon my recommendation, one of the prostate patients I observed who is the chief financial officer of a Fortune 500 company ingested the combination of noni, Ecomer®, Badmaev 269™, the proteolytic enzyme complex called Nutrizyme™, and the Chinese detoxifier Natura 401™. Electrodermal screening indicated that this five-product combination in predetermined appropriate dosages would reverse prostate cancer. After regular consumption of the combination, it did just that. In 60 days the CFO's symptomatology disappeared, and in 120 days his return to the urologist for a biopsy indicated that prostate cancer was totally gone," Dr. Kaltsas told me. "The man then had this biopsy report confirmed with a sonogram of his prostate, and no cancer showed.

"Amazing though it may seem, I have observed the same results from botanical use for those same patients I had already mentioned. These people are not supposed to get well from their cancers, but they do indeed by following the nutritional protocol that's known to work. The protocol may include six noni juice capsules taken three times a day if the patient's health problem is severe; ordinarily a maintenance dose is just six noni daily," says Dr. Harvey Kaltsas. "Noni together with the other formula elements do work well to eliminate many types of cancer."

Steven Schechter, N.D., Employs Noni for Different Conditions

Steven Schechter, N.D., of Encinitas, California, is an exponent of employing encapsulated noni. Dr. Schechter, who is dean of the Natural Healing Institute, a State-of-California-approved school in Encinitas, says: "I use noni to overcome several different conditions such as to reduce pain and cause it to be more manageable. Noni is well known in Hawaii as coming from the 'painkiller tree' or the 'headache bush' with its anti-inflammatory properties. I often combine noni juice capsules with other herbs such as feverfew for the treatment of headache. And noni offers endocrine-regulating effects for bringing down high blood pressure, correcting hypoglycemia, overcoming Type II (but not Type I) diabetes, and for creating a person's sense of well-being.

"Freeze-dried noni juice capsules from Hawaii help in the treatment of almost all cancers. And I've had great success in using it in powder form for relieving patients suffering from fibromyalgia," advises Dr. Steven Schechter. "The taking of noni capsules addresses all of the fibromyalgia concerns: fatigue, muscle and joint pain, and generalized inflammation. Because noni contains so many constituents—well over thirty—it provides numerous mechanisms of action. I love to use this product for it's so useful for multiple health problems."

Resources

For more information about noni and the therapy derived from ingesting capsules of this adaptogenic substance, contact the manufacturer and distributor, American Nutriceuticals, Inc., 205 North Orange Avenue, Suite 1N, Sarasota, Florida 34236; telephone toll free (888) 848-2548 or locally (941) 365-5592; fax (941) 366-5923; e-mail: amnutri@aol.com.

9

Medicinal Mushroom

Did you know that certain mushrooms are extremely safe to consume and definitely provide the user with high-quality healing for a variety of serious health problems? Listed in this healing category are those mushrooms belonging to the family of Polyporaceae (also known as Basidiomycotinae). Among these Polyporaceae species is *Coriolus versicolor*, which shows great biological activity for the betterment of mankind. Of all the world's nations, physicians in Germany are most knowledgeable about the use of mushrooms for their medicinal properties. The German holistic-type oncologists have become exponents of mushroom therapy, especially for the elimination of their disease specialty—cancer. These enlightened doctors are now teaching mushroom medicine to North American health professionals who are not locked into drug use, chemotherapy, radiation, and other toxic conventional cancer therapies. They have opened many North American minds to health-care methods offered in complementary and alternative medicine (CAM).

The primary oncological consultant for this book's information on German cancer therapies, Helmut Keller, M.D., of Nordhalben, Germany, has made mushroom medicine an integral part of his anticancer protocol. Dr. Helmut Keller has routinely added the medicinal mushroom *Coriolus versicolor* to his successful Carnivora® malignancy treatment program. Surprisingly, he sends to the United States for acquiring quantities of a certain superior brand of *Coriolus versicolor* medicinal mushroom called VPS®. It is supplied in the form of capsules by the JHS Natural Products Company of Eugene, Oregon (see this chapter's Resource section for the JHS post office address, e-mail address, website address, and telephone/fax numbers).

A Brief Primer on Mushrooms

Did you know that numbers of different fungi have for at least forty centuries been vital parts of mythology and medical practice around the world? Fungally derived phytochemicals find significance among peoples along the Pacific Rim (Japan and Thailand), on the Asian continent (China and Russia), and inside the Third World countries of darkest Africa (especially within the Yoruba tribe of southwestern Nigeria).

There are more than half a million varieties of fungi (with over 100,000 named species). Are you aware that mushroom fungi hold value for most European residents? They have always appreciated the gastronomic excellence of both the domestic- and wild-growing species. Gourmet cooks, especially French, Belgian, and Austrian chefs, consider mushrooms "flowers of the fall" and label them in their recipes with this loving appellation.

Have you taken note that mushrooms are the perfect food for staying trim, remaining healthy, and feeling a sense of well-being? Because mushrooms contain only insignificant amounts of fat—predominantly as unsaturated linoleic acid—eating them as a rule helps one to hold on to a well-functioning cardiovascular system and stay free of malignancy.

Are you aware that most inhabitants of the United States, Canada, Great Britain, Australia, and New Zealand are rather ignorant about mushrooms? These English-speaking populations, in fact, actually dislike or fear ingesting them, because of "fungophobia"—the view that mushrooms are associated with unsavory or poisonous fungi.

Do you have fungophobia? In contrast to your possible prejudice or general misinformation, be advised that mushrooms possess medicinal value far surpassing or at least on a par with such beneficial phytochemicals (usually labelled nutriceuticals) as oligomeric proanthocyanidines (OPCs), d-alpha tocopherol (natural vitamin E), thymus gland extract, coenzyme Q_{10}, olive leaf extract, and particular probiotics such as the homeostatic soil organisms (HSOs).

It's known that oncologist Friedrich Douwes, M.D., of Bad Aibling, Germany, recently received a particularly large shipment of VPS® *Coriolus versicolor* for his oral administration to patients in their fight against varieties of cancer. Dr. Douwes showed me his well-stocked dispensary at the St. Georg Hospital in Bad Aibling in which many encapsulated remedies are stored—VPS *Coriolus versicolor* among them. This medicinal mushroom is a main component in the Douwes anticancer protocol.

The Medicinal Mushroom Usage of Steven Bailey, N.D.

"Of all medicinal plants, *Coriolus versicolor* is one of the safest and most effective agents any doctor can use against chronic diseases. This mushroom places no metabolic demand on the liver or extenuating stress on the kidneys," says the American naturopathic doctor Steven Bailey, of Portland, Oregon. "So when one looks at treatment risks for all of the recognized phytochemical products, the *Coriolus versicolor* mushroom exhibits one of the lowest treatment imperilments for viral infection, malignant tumors, or immune system depression.

"I see the *Coriolus versicolor* product processed and distributed by the JHS Natural Products Company of Eugene, Oregon, as having a very high degree of reliability for boosting human and animal immune system function. The JHS brand-named mushroom product, VPS®, does this in ways that are beneficial not only for the body's surveillance or destruction of tumors but also as a protector against secondary infection," Dr. Bailey confirms. "The two immunologically active fractions of this therapeutic mushroom negate or decrease side effects connected with chemotherapy, surgery, and radiotherapy. And those fractions offset other chronic immune imbalances, including autoimmune diseases. Definitely I consider the VPS® brand of PSK *Coriolus versicolor* to be a potent immune system builder that's easy for the patients to ingest as capsules."

In private practice for twenty years, Dr. Bailey has taught courses in nutrition and pharmacognosy at the National College of Naturopathic Medicine in Portland. He has been using the *Coriolus versicolor* polysaccharide extract for six years to relieve such illnesses or traumas as hepatitis B and C, AIDS, herpes genitalis, cancer, general immune suppression, and postsurgical recovery. Usually Dr. Bailey doesn't administer the *Coriolus* polysaccharides as a single treatment agent; rather, it becomes part of his fairly comprehensive nutritional protocol.

"Of course, some cancer patients take *Coriolus versicolor* even while they engage in radiation treatment or chemotherapy," Dr. Baily advises. "Or the patients don't submit to chemotherapy or radiotherapy at all but rely, instead, exclusively on nutritional therapies with the mushroom as a main treatment ingredient. For example, one of my patients, Martha I., a thirty-four-year-old woman working in the health field, consulted me with a cancer spreading at two sites in her lungs. Orthodox treatment had been tried but no longer was effective. She discontinued her smoking of two cigarette packs a day and embarked on nutritional therapies. The nutrients included Martha's completing six months of taking *Coriolus versicolor*. After this half-year, radiological examination showed that all of her lung tumors had disappeared. Seeing her current progress, orthodox medicine probably would declare this patient to be cured."

CAM physicians tend to disagree with the concept of "curing" cancer. Their admonitions to this cancer patient would likely be that she should take the JHS *Coriolus versicolor* product for the rest of her life as a form of health insurance against the return of lung cancer. That is Dr. Steven Bailey's recommendation too.

Physical Characteristics of *Coriolus Versicolor*

Published in Japan since the 1970s, over 400 clinical studies have shown that a purified extract derived from the mushroom *Coriolus versicolor* offers strong benefits for the immune system. The VPS-branded extract from JHS Natural Products is a protein-bound polysaccharide preparation isolated from the mushroom's mycelia and fruiting bodies by use of hot water in a multistep procedure. After completion of the extraction process, the evolved solution is concentrated and dehydrated. The brownish mushroom powder remaining is encapsulated and ingested for its therapeutic effects.

Taken either alone or with conventional chemotherapy or radiotherapy for cancer, three or more grams per day of this brown-powdered extract, administered orally, results in antitumor activity. In vivo studies of rats and mice show that *Coriolus* polysaccharides work well against a variety of experimental animal cancers such as sarcoma, hepatoma, and fibrosarcoma.[1]

Coriolus versicolor goes by a number of botanical names, including *Trametes versicolor*,[2] *Boletus versicolor*, *Polyporus versicolor*,[3] and *Polystictus versicolor*,[4] and the common idiomatic attribution of "turkey tail." The fruiting bodies do resemble a fanned turkey tail, and the *versicolor* name comes from this mushroom being variously colored. In Japan it's called *kawaratake*, which means "mushroom by the river bank."[5] Among the common people in China, the fungus is referred to as *yun-zhi*, indicating that it's a cloud fungus and grows best in the rain.[6]

As an often-seen denizen of the woods populating the temperate zones of North America, Asia, and Europe, *Coriolus versicolor* possesses fan-shaped fruiting bodies that grow in overlapping clusters on dead trees. The mushroom's top portion is zoned, usually in shades of brown, white, gray, or blue, and it sports hairy bands. The underside of its cap is white and shows minute pores that do not discolor after scratching.[7]

Active Medicinal Components of the Mushroom

The mushroom's active medicinal components—biological response modifiers which are protein-bound polysaccharides—can be found in both the fungus's fruiting body and its mycelium (the vegetative stage).

Although these concentrated polysaccharide extracts are sold under a variety of trade names in North America and Asia such as VPS®, they are most commonly referred to by the Japanese as water-soluble "Polysaccharide Kureha" or Polysaccharide K (commonly referred to as PSK by those informed patients using *Coriolus versicolor*). PSK contains the main components of the cancer fighter -1,4- and -1,6- glucans with -1,3- and -1,6- linkages.[8,9] Also the mushroom contains other medicinal components of secondary importance.[10]

All of these potent but safely used medicinal components are reported as particularly effective against stomach (gastric) cancer,[11,12,13,14,15] uterine cancer,[16] colon cancer, and lung cancer.[17]

As clinically and anecdotally reported below, the mushroom extract additionally works well against colorectal cancer, prostate cancer, breast cancer, and liver cancer.

PSK Acts Alone Against Colorectal Cancer

Publishing in *Cancer Immunology and Immunotherapy,* no less than eleven oncological researchers representing six prestigious medical schools in Japan conducted a randomized double-blind trial on 111 patients who had colorectal cancer. After they had undergone surgical operations for their cancers, 56 patients were given PSK alone as an active treatment substance, and 55 other postsurgical patients merely received a placebo.

Comparing the two groups, these eleven medical researchers advised, "There is significant prolongation of disease-free periods for patients with colorectal cancer who took PSK. Additionally, polymorphonuclear leukocytes from patients treated with *Coriolus versicolor* showed remarkable enhancement in their activities, such as random and/or chemotactic locomotion, and phagocytosis. In conclusion, PSK was useful as a maintenance therapy for patients after their curative surgical operations for colorectal cancer. The beneficial effects were probably due to the activation of leukocyte functions as one of the many biological-response-modifying activities induced by PSK (VPS®)."[18]

Kenneth Bock, M.D., Observes PSK Boosts NK Cells

"Because it increases natural killer [NK] cell activity, I think of using *Coriolus versicolor* mainly when I'm confronted with a patient suffering from cancer or a viral infection," says Kenneth A. Bock, M.D., medical director of two holistic medical clinics, one located in Rhinebeck, New York, and the other in Albany, New York. "This mushroom is one of the main medicinal compounds I use to boost a diminished blood reading which records NK activity. PSK does produce a marked improvement in NK cell function and number, something I monitor by blood testing. If the blood reading is low, my patient takes greater amounts of PSK capsules. And, although it's an expensive and sophisticated assay, I repeat my NK cell testing inside of a month or two. In a number of patients, I've seen some nice blood test improvements.

"Before consulting me, a few patients with advanced metastatic cancer show NK cell activities of only 2 or 3 minute units (m/u). Normal measurement for the laboratory I employ is between 20 and 50 m/u. By my using PSK for most of these patients, I have observed their NK cells increasing into the normal range. They then experience an improved prognosis," says Dr. Bock. "I can illustrate what I'm saying by providing a before-and-after patient case history plus the literature that backs my claim.[19,20,21]

"Here is a white, married male named Marty E., sixty years old, working as a computer consultant, who originally had been followed medically for hypertension, hyperlipidemia, and arteriosclerosis, during 1995. He also exhibited laryngeal polyps which were cancerous. Marty received radiation therapy as a follow-up to the surgery performed to remove these polyps," points out Dr. Bock.

"At the time of surgery, a CT scan to his pelvis was negative for cancer metastasis to the prostate. But later, in April 1997, my patient did show an elevated PSA [prostate-specific antigen] and underwent an additional medical workup, including biopsy. Workup results indicated his true diagnosis, which was prostate cancer. His blood test showed diminished natural killer cell activity at the level of 6 m/u. Still, Marty wanted no conventional therapy for the prostate cancer," Dr. Bock tells me. "So I started him on alternative medical therapies for prostate cancer and to improve his deficient NK cell activity. *Coriolus versicolor* was a definite part of his treatment regimen.

"Within two months, the patient's NK [natural killer] cell activity elevated to 18 m/u. And two months after that his NK cell activity increased to a normal 31 m/u. Now the man is doing well physically, and he tells me he feels great! I would say that this type of response to the VPS brand of PSK therapy is usual; the patient's quality of life does improve dramatically and he or she feels a sense of well-being," Dr. Bock states.

Animal Studies of *Coriolus Versicolor*

Animal studies investigating the efficacy of *Coriolus versicolor* indicate it has marked immune-system-enhancing activity and a broad antineoplastic scope. It prolongs the survival time of irradiated (cancer-induced) mice by stimulating phagocytic activity of macrophages and improving the functions of the reticuloendothelial system.[22] For another rodent type of disease, cyclophosphamide-induced granulocytopenia in mice, PSK caused a significant increase in granulocyte production.[23] Also it restored antibody (IgG) production in mice bearing sarcoma 180, but not in normal mice.[24]

PSK acts directly against tumor cells as well as indirectly in the host to boost cellular immunity. The following is a listing of cancers for which it is known to be efficacious in animals: adenosarcoma, fibrosarcoma, mastocytoma, plasmacytoma, melanoma, sarcoma, carcinoma, mammary cancer, colon cancer, and lung cancer.[25] Indeed, injection of the PSK compound at one tumor site shows tumor growth inhibition at other sites, thus helping to prevent metastasis.[26] Moreover, its antitumor activity increases when PSK is administered in combination with radiation, chemotherapy, or immunotherapy. Giving the polysaccharide substance in 10 percent or less of rat feeds does suppress carcinogen-induced rodent cancers of the colon, esophagus, breast, and lung.[27]

PSK demonstrates antiviral activity and may be effective against human immunodeficiency virus (HIV) infection by modifying the viral receptor or by stopping it from binding with lymphocytes.[28] Another mechanism by which PSK shows general antiviral activity is through the stimulation of interferon production.[29]

On ingestion, whole *Coriolus versicolor* lowers serum cholesterol in animals.[30] In combination with the herb *Astragalus membranaceus* Bunge, it enhances neutrophil function and speeds recovery in rabbits suffering from burns.[31] A powdered extract of PSK from the 70 percent ethanolic tincture of this species tested in rats by injection in a Hippocratic screening of higher fungi did demonstrate mild tranquilizing and diuretic effects.[32]

PSK Is Supportive of Chemotherapy and Radiotherapy

Providing strong benefits for the immune system when given alone, *Coriolus versicolor* works even more supportively against cancer after it's applied with chemotherapy and/or radiotherapy. In fact, out of 200 adjunctive phytochemicals screened for antitumor activity by Japanese researchers in 1971, PSK was selected as the best adjunctive treatment.

The researchers suggested that this medicinal mushroom seemed to protect the immune system's activity from being suppressed by prolonged use of chemotherapy drugs and by the toxic processes of the cancer itself. Added to that finding, a ten-year study of 185 patients with lung cancer showed that combining PSK with radiation therapy produced "satisfactory" tumor shrinkage and better survival rates for patients with Stage I cancer (39 percent) and Stage II cancer (22 percent) compared against those patients with Stage I cancer (16 percent) and Stage II cancer (5 percent) who did not receive this combination of therapies.[33]

Reporting the above study in another, more exacting way: From 1976 to 1985, 185 patients with non–small cell lung cancer at Stages I, II, and III were treated with definitive radiotherapy in Gunma University Hospital at the Gunma University School of Medicine in Maebashi, Japan. The long-term survivors were analyzed carefully. Those who had received *Coriolus versicolor* as adjuvant treatment showed more satisfactory tumor shrinkage and their five-year survival rate was better than those patients not receiving PSK. That is, PSK patients with Stage I or II disease showed up with 39 percent survival; PSK patients with Stage III cancer had 22 percent survival. Comparing these survivors with the Stage I and Stage II non-PSK group, we see that these non-PSK patients had only 16 percent and 5 percent survival, respectively. The non-PSK Stage III patients had no survivors.[34]

In Japan, the standard adjuvant treatment after resection of gastric cancer is a combination of two cytotoxic drugs, intravenous mitomycin plus oral fluorouracil. As a clinical test, the protein-bound polysaccharide PSK was added to this standard chemotherapy for 262 randomly assigned patients. Half received *Coriolus versicolor* and half took the usual chemotherapy alone after all of them had undergone what the Japanese label "curative" gastrectomy. During a minimum follow-up of five years (ranging from five to seven years), the clinical testing took place at forty-six institutions in central Japan.

PSK improved the cancer patients' five-year disease-free rate at 70.7 percent versus 59.4 percent in a standard treatment group (p = 0.047). And it improved their five-year survival rate at 73.0 percent versus 60.0 percent, (p = 0.044) as well. The two regimens had only slight toxic effects, consisting of nausea, leukopenia, and liver function impairment. There were no significant differences between the groups. The treatments were clinically well tolerated and compliance of patients was good. In their paper published in *Lancet*, the researchers concluded, "Addition of PSK to adjuvant chemotherapy with mitomycin and fluorouracil is beneficial as treatment after curative gastrectomy."[35]

Between January 1980 and December 1990, 222 operable breast

cancer patients with vascular invasion in their tumors and/or in their metastatic lymph nodes were randomized into three treatment groups. Group one received a combination of toxic therapies, what the researchers labeled "FEMP" (5-fluorouracil, cyclophosphamide, mitomycin C, and prednisone). Group two received FEMP plus LMS (levamisole). Group three received FEMP plus PSK.

The seven Japanese researchers concluded: "Immunochemotherapy using PSK improved the prognosis of patients having operable breast cancer with vascular invasion. . . . The prognosis of the FEMP + PSK group tended to be better than that of the FEMP group. FEMP + PSK is better because of its usefulness including good compliance."[36]

Twenty-eight patients suffering from acute leukemia who had achieved complete remission participated in a clinical trial. Starting in September 1976, half of these patients entering the chemo-PSK immunotherapy group received the medicinal mushroom *Coriolus versicolor*, and half entering the strictly chemotherapy group did not. To retain the patients' remission, all of them received three courses of the chemotherapy combination of cytotoxics consisting of 40 units/kg/day of neocarzinostatin; 0.8–1.6 mg/kg/day of cytosine arabinoside; 0.6–0.8 mg/kg/day of daunorubicin; and 0.8–1.6 mg/kg/day of prednisolone on days one to four for acute nonlymphocytic leukemia, and 0.04 mg/kg/day of vincristine on day one; 0.6–0.8 mg/kg/day of daunorubicin; and 0.8–1.6 mg/kg/day of prednisolone on days one to four for acute lymphocytic leukemia.

The durations of complete remission and survival in the chemo-PSK immunotherapy group (receiving PSK) showed significant prolongation compared to that of the strictly chemotherapy group (not receiving PSK). The median duration of complete remission for this PSK group was thirty-six weeks and that for the non-PSK group was twenty-five weeks. The average survival time from diagnosis of the PSK group was twenty-one months and that of the non-PSK group was twelve months.[37]

Tori Hudson, N.D., Uses *Coriolus Versicolor*

"The only condition I've been using *Coriolus versicolor* for is breast cancer, Stage II and above, in which the patients have been actively receiving chemotherapy. If they are just starting their chemotherapy, I've added PSK. When the patients are finished with their chemotherapy I've continued the PSK. This procedure is followed in accordance with my understanding of the few research articles I've read relative to breast cancer patients and PSK. My intention is to keep the breast cancer patient taking *Coriolus versicolor* for a total of five years. But I've been using the mushroom for only three years now," says naturopathic physician Tori Hudson, N.D.

"I have just begun using PSK for a man who is facing the recurrence of gastric cancer. He's had a full gamut of therapies and still shows elevated cancer markers which his oncologist finds untreatable. The patient was referred to me for some alternative cancer therapy because conventional oncology has nothing more to use on him," says Dr. Hudson. "My impression is that patients taking *Coriolus versicolor* are experiencing less side effects from chemotherapy such as diminished fatigue, less nausea (but not less hair loss), and more stable white blood cell counts. I have not measured the natural killer cell counts."

A Patient's Experience with Liver Cancer Reduction

A sixty-four-year-old electrical engineer in Tyler, Texas, Allen G., had been treated for liver cancer for six years. In the beginning stages of his malignancy, he took chemotherapy, which eventually proved to do no good. And the oncologist offered him absolutely nothing more as treatment, not even personal care to accomplish a better quality of life for himself—no improved diet, nutrients, exercise, meditation—just nothing at all.

"That doctor was the most negative man I ever met," said Mr.

G. "After the chemo failed, he threw up his hands, shrugged his shoulders, wished me good luck, and said there was nothing else he could do. And surgery couldn't be performed either, because the consulting surgeon saw that the tumor was wrapped around my vena cava blood vessel."

The patient replied to his oncologist, "I totally reject what you are telling me. I do not accept that nothing can be done to affect the outcome of this disease."

When the doctor said, "Well, I know what I'm talking about when it comes to cancer. I'm a scientist."

Allen G. shot back, "Yes, but you're not God!"

Even with being abandoned by his oncologist, today the patient is healthy once again after utilizing alternative methods of healing, most especially by his self-administration of oral *Coriolus versicolor*. Mr. G.'s tumor, which had been situated on the left lobe of the liver, was sized at 10 cm by 7 cm and by the longitudinal measurement of 9 cm. Now, after he has been taking capsules of VPS from the JHS Natural Products Company, the tumor has shrunk to 5 cm by 4 cm by 3 cm (longitudinally). The patient had learned about *Coriolus versicolor* from contacting Medline on the Internet. By digging into the World Wide Web, he has saved himself. Remarkably, the volume of Mr. G.'s liver cancer has reduced to less than 10 percent of its original size, from 630 cm^3 down to 60 cm^3. And his carcinoembryonic antigen (CEA) cancer marker has improved dramatically as well, dropping from 296 to 97.9.

Today, after four years, Mr. G. still swallows VPS, those brownish-colored mushroom capsules, which he intends to take for the rest of his life. He is well versed in the efficacy of *Coriolus versicolor*, having read nearly four hundred studies about PSK that he printed out from the Internet.

Resources

The VPS brand of *Coriolus versicolor* (or PSK) is furnished without prescription by JHS Natural Products, P.O. Box 50398, Eugene, Oregon 97405; telephone toll free (888) 330-4691 or (541) 344-1396; fax (541) 344-3107; e-mail: jhsinfo@jhsnp.com; website: www.jhsnp.com.

10

Induced Remission Therapy

Among the active cancer therapies that this book's oncology consultant, Helmut G. Keller, M.D., of Nordhalben, Germany, cites as highly successful is Induced Remission Therapy® (IRT). In a self-published treatise on his personal life's work in restoring cancer patients to health, Dr. Helmut Keller states that he considers IRT equal in importance for cancer victims to his own invention, Carnivora®. When available, he acquires a supply of the IRT vaccine from its developer and employs this antiserum as part of his treatment protocol for people with almost any kind of malignancy. Other German doctors, having discovered its usefulness, also apply IRT as a part of their anticancer protocols.

Induced Remission Therapy® has been conceived, developed, legally administered, and is currently taught to physicians worldwide by a forty-year-old, Australian-born, Jewish medical genius of Egyptian ancestry. This treatment is available today as invented and developed by research physician, oncologist/immunologist Samir Chachoua, M.B., B.S. He is licensed as a medical doctor in Australia, China, England, anywhere that licensure reciprocity prevails in the British Commonwealth (Scotland, Wales, Ireland, etc.), Mexico, India, and Guatemala. (Dr. Chachoua's M.B. stands for an Australian medical school's

Bachelor of Medicine degree and his B.S. stands for the Australian medical school's Bachelor of Surgery degree. The M.B. and B.S. are doctoral degrees similar to those offered to medical graduates in England and other countries of the United Kingdom.) The M.B. and B.S. are of similar or higher equivalency to the American M.D. (Doctor of Medicine) degree.

Induced Remission Therapy® has evolved out of the loving memory Dr. Sam Chachoua holds for his father, Dr. Isaac Chachoua, who succumbed to the highly lethal bone cancer multiple myeloma. Dr. Isaac Chachoua had practiced medicine in Australia. Even while he was facing death, his teenage son was performing medical research at Australia's Peter McCallum Cancer Institute to stem the father's illness. (Dr. Sam graduated from medical school at age eighteen and presented his cancer therapy findings to a prestigious medical forum at age nineteen.)

Dr. Sam's numerous discoveries connected with IRT did not arrive in time to save his father. But now, these remarkably unprecedented oncological breakthroughs are reversing cancer in better than nine out of ten patients who manage to access the treatment. It is available in North America, some Caribbean countries, the Bahamas, Central America, and South America, especially in Mexico, Guatemala, and Argentina. IRT is used extensively as one of the more significant German cancer therapies in the various German-speaking nations. Gradually IRT is being picked up and used by American physicians who are willing to invest time in learning about it.

Dr. Sam Chachoua Wins Suit Against Cedars-Sinai Medical Center

On August 15, 2000, in Los Angeles, a United States District Court with the Honorable Margaret M. Morrow, judge presiding, awarded to plaintiff Samir Chachoua, M.B., B.S., $10,111,250 in damages as a result of his legal action against the renowned Los Angeles–based Cedars-Sinai Medical Center and its department chief of immunology as defendants. In this unpublished Civil Case number 97-5595, the Cedars-Sinai Medical Center, University of California, Los Angeles, School of Medicine, Los Angeles, California, and Eric S. Daar, M.D., director of the Cedars-Sinai AIDS and Immune Disorder Center, Division of Infectious Diseases, were unanimously judged by a jury of eight to have failed to return proprietary anticancer and anti-AIDS vaccine cultures (IRT) to Dr. Sam Chachoua, thereby breaching its contract with him. This award was won as well because the jury found that Cedars-Sinai under the aegis of Dr. Eric Daar refused to publish the results of successful anticancer safety and efficacy tests it had conducted on Induced Remission Therapy® with appropriate credit to Samir Chachoua. It should be noted, however, that the court granted the defendants a new trial.

It is not known why the defendants failed to fulfill their contract with Dr. Chachoua or omitted any publication of positive findings on his IRT. It is known, however, that Cedars-Sinai has patented its own version of the plaintiff's IRT program. The treatment not only has validity against cancer, but also is proven effective for acquired immunodeficiency syndrome (AIDS) and heart disease. And Dr. Daar, claiming IRT to be his original work, did publish an article together with four colleagues in the 1996 issue, volume 12, no. 16, of *AIDS Research and Human Retroviruses*, issued by the medical journal publisher Mary Ann Liebert, Inc. By this publication, Dr. Daar and his colleagues appear to take credit for Dr. Chachoua's discovery that autoimmune disease stimulates antibodies that cross-react with HIV Type 1 infectivity.

IRT offers applications for eliminating numbers of diseases by addressing their causes and the regeneration of tissue such as new cardiac valves, brain cells, and much more. IRT brings about cellular restoration for diabetes, asthma, cardiovascular diseases, chronic fatigue syndrome, immune dysfunction, fibromyalgia, Gulf War syndrome, Parkinson's disease, Alzheimer's disease, and amyotrophic lateral sclerosis. (Please see court testimony below on the efficacy of Dr. Samir Chachoua's IRT for the elimination of AIDS, chronic fatigue syndrome, fibromyalgia, immune system dysfunction, and heart disease given by witnesses under oath in Federal District Court.)

Most of all, Induced Remission Therapy® possesses everactive cancer–reversing properties. The treatment achieves its healing effects with the use of vaccines prepared by means of Dr. Samir Chachoua's laboratory methods and clinical procedures.

Four Patients with Cancer Who Responded to IRT

• Patient One. Clinical application of IRT was rendered to a young woman, Rose C., whose brain tumor had previously failed to respond to both radiation therapy and chemotherapy. Medical staff who had treated her at the University of California Medical Center, Los Angeles, did not expect Ms. C. to survive past 1996. Inasmuch as she has undertaken IRT for the past six years now, it turns out that they were wrong. The patient's tumors have been persistently regressing. She is alive, happy, and productive.

• Patient Two. The lung cancer of Doris M. responded exceedingly well to a limited supply of Dr. Chachoua's vaccines. Her liver metastases have shrunk too. Because the IRT vaccine supply ran out as a result of the Cedars-Sinai debacle when they held back Dr. Chachoua's primary cultures for making a new batch, the disease has recurred. Presently Ms. M.'s life is threatened by the recurrence of her prior lung cancer.

• Patient Three. With a breast cancer tumor that had doubled in size within just a few weeks, Janet I. was in difficulty for her life, especially since some axillary lymph nodes (in her left armpit) were indicating the presence of cancer. Also, a chronic cough suggested lung involvement. But six years ago Ms. I. began on IRT and improvement set in. From then on her lungs have remained clear and free of cancer. There has been no growth in metastasized lymph nodes or the primary breast tumor.

• Patient Four. Althea M. was struck with breast cancer and melanoma about half a dozen years ago. She became wheelchair bound as a result of leg and back involvement with the disease. Upon the woman's electing to receive IRT a year after her diagnosis, Ms. M.'s body response to the treatment was immediate. She remains disease-free today.

An Abstracted Overview of Induced Remission Therapy

Since cancer cellular pathology is not readily recognizable by the human immune system, it is necessary to change the appearance of cancer cells so that they may be immunologically attacked. Induced Remission Therapy® attempts and usually succeeds in making the malignancy look like something that is easy for the body to destroy. IRT takes a cancer cell that the body ordinarily cannot see and tags it with certain proteins that alter the cancer to look like a cold or the flu. These kinds of common infections the immune system is able to attack and fight off.

Further to this end, IRT provides the required immune response to battle against the appearance of that new disease such as a cold or influenza. If a person's immune system identifies cancer as resembling one of the more common forms of illnesses, it will quickly attack and reject the deadly disease. (Of course, this description is a very gross simplification of a highly complex mechanism.) IRT is based on a heretofore unknown immune response which is isolated from people who are resistant to cancer. These cancer-resistant persons are those who are affected by autoimmune diseases such as rheumatoid arthritis, thyroiditis, autoallergy, thrombocytopenia, autoimmune hemolytic anemia, systemic lupus erythematosus, Crohn's disease, and more. (Who could have predicted that there exists some benefit to suffering from one of these serious health problems? Cancer seldom affects a person exhibiting an autoimmune illness.)

The advantage of inheriting an autoimmune response—even an adverse one—is that it penetrates the cells, including cancer cells. The agent required to change the appearance of a cancer cell is acquired by use of Dr. Chachoua's technique, and that agent is then planted into the cancer cell nucleus (its heart and brain). Then the body develops an altered immune response that goes into the cancer cell and genetically corrects the disease. In effect, IRT makes cancer look like something that the body's immunity will attack and then provides that very same immune response to fight the disease.

This is what Dr. Chachoua does for patients seeking his services for the reversal of cancer. He does not ordinarily consult with patients. Instead, he creates a vaccine that becomes the therapeutic agent for an individual and then dispenses it to the person's attending physician for use as treatment. One may be surprised to learn that the Australian physician does not sell this vaccine; rather, Dr. Chachoua offers training in his treatment technology to practicing physicians so that they may implement it for patients.

IRT is available in most Latin American countries. Where the law allows utilization of the vaccine in the United States and Canada under the Health Freedoms Act, and a patient's medical doctor accepts training and responsibility in producing and administering the vaccine, Dr. Chachoua makes it available to that health professional. This Australian-born medical inventor takes no fee for such teaching of administration technique and vaccine supply.

For basic IRT, which entails producing vaccine by use of the measles or mumps virus or an animal virus, the cost is just a few hundred dollars. More sophisticated autogenous vaccines designed to genetically affect cancer cells for a longer-lasting response may run into the thousands of dollars. To replace stem cells using therapeutic extracts such as a bone marrow transplant, a vaccine of this type may run into the hundreds of thousands of dollars (but such treatment often is covered by health insurance). If health insurance fails to pay vaccine costs and the patient cannot afford the related, elevated treatment fees, Dr. Sam Chachoua's American patient-formed charitable foundation named Save-a-Life Foundation, located in Boulder, Colorado, does supplement certain expenditures for individuals requiring the more sophisticated Induced Remission Therapy®. The primary purpose of Save-a-Life Foundation is to raise funds for further medical research on IRT, but sometimes it helps ill patients who need financial assistance.

The Applications Protocol of IRT for Cancer

During fourteen years he expended in medical research and his payout of no less than $12 million from his personal funds, Dr. Samir Chachoua uncovered an immense amount of information about the human immune system's response mechanism to physiological attack by foreign invaders both singularly and as a complex. For example, one of the medical realities that Dr. Chachoua learned is that fat cells not only encapsulate infections to provide an immune barrier to their spread, but fat also acts as a shield against cancer antigens and disease fragment processing. He observed that hairy tumor fat tissue forms a base for anticancer vaccines. The encapsulation mechanism of fat cells allows for a metabolic immune response.

Metabolic immune response (MIR) works best when the invader or irritant is overwhelming, when many forms of the invader exist, and/or when a nonspecific immune response is present at the time of the attack. To illustrate how MIR works, try to see the entire mechanism as an automobile running at top speed on gasoline. Here the gasoline is an invader of the auto; the faster this car is run, the quicker will be the breakdown of the invader. It gets used up. The same thing happens with cancer; the greater the MIR, the faster a malignancy dissipates.

Reflecting back to that period about two hundred years ago when cancer was considered to be infectious, Dr. Sam observed that patients undergoing spontaneous remission for cancer did so in response to the presence of an acute infection. In contrast, a chronic infection actually can cause cancer. That's because an aggressive and acute infection stimulates the MIR in cancer cells so that they commit preprogrammed suicide (apoptosis) and melt away.

Dr. Sam States that Cancer Is Not a Disease

Dr. Sam Chachoua describes a cancer cell not as a mindless beast resulting from random mutation as is the current concept, but rather as the stimulating agent for a weakened immune response. Cancer serves an important purpose demanded by nature to bring about invader encapsulation, metabolic elimination, and disease attenuation. Dr. Sam suggests that people must become aware of a startling life-extension fact: As cancer has increased among the world's populations just a century ago from one person in three hundred to the current incidence of every third person today, there has also been a simultaneous increase in human life expectancy. The decline in death from microorganism infections did not begin with antibiotics, vaccines, or excellent hygiene but has become the mirror image of the increase in cancer. Thus, cancer cells do serve nature's purpose. They enable the human physiology to achieve a sustained, long-term MIR (metabolic immune response) which inhibits and destroys infectious organisms and allows approximately two out of three people residing in Western industrialized countries to live longer.

Dr. Sam states convincingly that cancer is not a disease; it is a preprogrammed cellular response to the onset of disease. Every one of the 80 trillion cells in a human body contains this programming from its birth. And each form of cancer behaves in the same way from one person to the next. Realize that:

- Almost all cancers occur in clusters of specific age groups.
- They pass through the blood-brain barrier.
- Cancer cells are powerful immune stimulants.
- They produce anticancer compounds such as intraserum.
- Cancer cells carry messages for causing drug resistance and metastases.
- When one type of cancer is eliminated, another kind often arises in its place.
- Particular cancers strike repeatedly at the same class of people duplicating race, geographic areas, environmental factions, and more.

There is no denying, for instance, that bowel cancer exhibits similar growth patterns in identical areas and times of spread. All of this happens because of preprogramming within the cancer cells, and that is a primary discovery made by Dr. Sam Chachoua.

Further to his findings, Dr. Sam declares that cancer cells survive in chaos. They arise for only short periods to hold and restrain a pathological invader until the body can put up an appropriate immune response. Then the cancer cells commit apoptotic suicide and leave the body as waste products.

In tetanus-injecting experiments on laboratory rats simultaneously given cancer by Dr. Chachoua, the rats did not die from tetanus when ordinarily they should have succumbed in days. The encapsulation of tetanus organisms by cancer cells protected the animals against coming down with the infection. The same thing happens in plants. Crown gall disease is a plant cancer that protects the plant against infection with *Agrobacterium tumefaciens.*

Tagging Cancer Cells for Immune System Recognition

Because the immune system fails to recognize a cancer cell as pathologic, its dangerous characteristics remain hidden from any immune response. As mentioned, tagging the cancer cell with a common infection such as measles, mumps, the flu, or a cold virus causes antigens to be expressed on its cellular surface for up to three weeks. This gives time—a window of opportunity—for the immune response to rush in and attack the tagged cancer. If the cancer cell manages to subjugate the common infection, the infection's antigens cease their expression, and the immune system becomes blind to the cancer once again.

By the unique technique of his discovery, Dr. Chachoua's Induced Remission Therapy® optimizes an immune response within the time window. IRT seeks to correct disease at the genetic blueprint level and targets the cause of disease and then corrects cell damage at this same gene level. Cancers are allowed to then activate differentiation cycles or fulfill a programmed apoptotic cell death (they commit their preprogammed suicide). Diseased tissue is removed as waste, and there is a return to normal structure without trauma or toxicity in the body system or organ. By this manner, cancer is disposed of effectively. Remission takes place.

Testimony Under Oath About IRT Efficacy
for Other Illnesses

Testifying under oath on August 3, 2000, in United States District Court, Central District of California, Michael P. of Denver, Colorado, a retired biomedical electronic technician who had worked for Medtronic, Inc., an open heart surgery technical company, told of having to leave his job because of chronic fatigue. Fatigue became overwhelming for him, and he tested positive with human immunodeficiency virus (HIV). Mr. P. appeared in the courtroom on behalf of the plaintiff. Under questioning on the witness stand he stated:

"I was diagnosed with full-blown AIDS in 1996. HIV is the preliminary stages of AIDS. AIDS is when HIV becomes to a point in your life where it causes you to be fatigued, causes your immune system to react adversely to opportunistic infections and stresses," said Mr. P. "Ultimately it kills you! I was also diagnosed with pneumocystis pneumonia and unable to work. It was then that I began to take the vaccines [Dr. Chachoua's IRT].

"I took another series of vaccines in 1997, and since then I have taken more vaccines," Michael P. testified. "Now I feel great, and blood tests I took at Cedars-Sinai Medical Center show results consistent with my good feelings. So from 1996 to 2000 I have been taking Dr. Chachoua's vaccines and my health has improved dramatically."

Earlier the same day, Terry D. of Atlanta, Georgia, testified too. Mr. D. is now retired from his business management position at the American Telephone and Telegraph Co. because of being affected by AIDS. Under oath, Mr. D. stated:

"Through my Atlanta physician, Dr. Richardson, since 1996 I have been receiving Dr. Chachoua's vaccines that come from Mexico [from Baja California near the city of Ensenada]. Within one week of taking Dr. Chachoua's vaccines my T-helper cell count rose from 168 to 962, and my PCR [polymerase chain reaction, which when elevated indicates infection with HIV] dropped from 74,000 to 12,200. Those are significant results in the improvement of my fight against AIDS," states Terry D. "Dr. Chachoua's vaccines put me into remission. I am here [as a plaintiff's witness] because I represent the victims who have AIDS."

As another plaintiff's witness appearing on the same date, August 3, 2000, computer technician George N. from Wixom, Michigan, stated: "I was receiving treatment for chronic fatigue syndrome, immune dysfunction, and fibromyalgia in September and October 1998. Before taking IRT I was very sick, bedridden. But then the vaccines made me feel very well." The IRT worked well for him so that Mr. N. currently no longer suffers from the several conditions that had him symptomatic with illnesses.

In a public trial document, the heart problem patient fifty-nine-year-old Arthur M., owner of the Michigan Corporation, United Technologies International, testified on the public record. As another plaintiff's witness, on the trial's third day, of what turned out to be eight days of courtroom action, Mr. M. described how his heart difficulty responded to Induced Remission Therapy® :

"I had been huffing and puffing and had to be carried up and down stairs. So it was suggested to me by my electrical engineering colleague, Walter [R.], that I go and get some of Dr. Sam Chachoua's vaccines. So I flew out to see him [in Baja California, Mexico] and had a heart attack on the plane. I was in really bad shape," says Mr. M. "I was very skeptical when I walked into his office, and I felt like leaving.

"But I stayed, thank God, and Dr. Chachoua started working with me at 2:30 in the morning by giving me a shot [an injection with IRT vaccine]. That was on Labor Day of September 1996, and there he gave me six shots over six days. My whole life changed on that third day—I felt better—a big change. By the sixth day I felt an unusual amount of strength," affirms Arthur M. "I had blockage in five arteries, three of them were blocked by 87 percent, 62 percent, and 31 percent. But now [after IRT], I can do all kinds of things I could never do before. I do landscaping now but before I couldn't even lift a rake. Today I do it all. I just finished laying out 750 bags of fertilizer. I had gone to see Dr. Chachoua about my cardiovascular condition. Since then, I took an electrocardiogram six months later, and it showed total reversals of my heart and artery conditions."

As stated, at the conclusion of this legal action with a jury verdict rendered on August 10, 2000, but filed in the United States District Court of California on August 15, 2000, the verdict confirmed the efficacy of IRT. The suit had been brought by Samir Chachoua, M.B., S.B., as plaintiff, against Cedars-Sinai Medical Center, Division of Infectious Diseases, University of California, Los Angeles, School of Medicine, Los Angeles, California 90048, and Eric S. Daar, M.D. The jury awarded to Dr. Samir Chachoua $10,111,250 to pay for recovery and/or restoration of primary cultures, vaccines, sera, and antisera which had been taken from him and never returned by the defendants.

By their verdict, the California jury affirmed that cures for cancer, AIDS, and other illnesses are at hand if only the Chachoua-supplied work product lost by Cedars-Sinai Medical Center can be reassembled by Dr. Samir Chachoua. He is currently hard at work restoring his material to productive amounts so that people's lives may be saved by their doctors who take the training necessary for the administration of Induced Remission Therapy®.

Resources

For further information about Induced Remission Therapy® (IRT) or to speak with Dr. Samir Chachoua directly, for open-minded holistic-oriented physicians to take oncological/immunological training from him, to acquire a supply of Dr. Chachoua's cancer-reversing vaccine, or to enter a Mexican or Guatemalan hospital as a patient to receive IRT, there are several national or international resources to contact:

• Get in touch with Dr. Samir Chachoua's Los Angeles–based secretary, Carol A. Barber, 4318 Glenroe Avenue, Apt #2, Marina Del Rey, California 90292; telephone (310) 373-1000; fax (310) 306-1177; no e-mail is available for Ms. Barber or Dr. Chachoua.

• Make inquiry to Dr. Sam Chachoua's sponsoring medical foundation, the International Health News (IHN), 1320 Point Street, Victoria, British Columbia, Canada V8K 1A5; telephone (250) 384-2524; the IHN website: http://www. yourhealthbase. com; e-mail: health@pinc.com; International Health News is a newsletter published by Hans R. Larsen. A compilation of its abstracts and research reports are published annually in a 200-page yearbook ISSN 1203-1933 or as an online e-book which is readable with the freely downloaded Adobe Acrobat Reader 4.0.

• Pull up and study the website for Biotechnologies International, a research organization located at Biotechnologies North America, 3001 North Rocky Point Drive, Suite 200, Tampa, Florida 33607 U.S.A.; telephone (813) 281-5460; fax (813) 289-7748. This organization is investigating everything known about the efficacy and/or legitimacy of Dr. Samir Chachoua's Induced Remission Therapy®. The website of Biotechnologies International is http//www.biotechnologies international.com.

• One might attempt to reach Dr. Sam Chachoua at his part-time residence in Baja California, Mexico, by telephone and/or fax. His single-line fax/phone number is (011) 526-630-8507. It is rare to find Dr. Sam at his Mexican home but he usually does respond to receiving a fax.

In the United States, you can leave a voicemail message at Dr. Sam's Southern California business office by phoning (310) 229-5275. Or you can reach Dr. Sam directly through his California attorney's e-mail address. Contact attorney Henry Ng at Nglaw@hotmail.com.

11

Cancer Marker Tests

Writing in his book *The Insecurity of Freedom* (1966), medical ethicist Abraham J. Heschel (1907 to 1972) advises: "The patient must not be defined as a client who contracts with a physician for service; he is a human being entrusted to the cure of a physician."

In the presence of end-stage cancer there may be needless suffering caused by indifference to the patient's terminal condition. Registered nurse Nancy Hassett Dahm, author of *Mind, Body and Soul: A Guide to Living with Cancer* (referenced at www.cancerbook.com), states that "some physicians treat terminal cancer patients as 'write-offs' and use them as proving grounds for their 'pet procedures.' Most hospitals cannot adequately care for end-stage cancer patients because of a pervasive lack of knowledge and reliance on antiquated treatments [and viable cancer marker tests] which have long outlived their effectiveness. I've seen too much needless suffering in cancer treatment and an appalling lack of attention paid to the very essence of what makes us human. While the medical establishment tries to 'treat and cure' cancer, an epidemic of preventable patient misery is happening right before our eyes. It doesn't have to be this way."

Sometimes the cancer patient teetering on the edge of death

is lost sight of as a human being who requires the ultimate in care and concern. Such lack of caring may be indicated by a certain insufficiency in the recording of his or her cancer markers by an attending or consulting physician. My observation is that such a negative circumstance—inadequate laboratory or clinical testing—is seldom the situation in the cancer specialists of Western Europe.

Holistic oncologists in Germany are aware of the cancer patient's need to restore immunity. They realize that a malfunctional immune system is the main reason anyone is brought into a cancerous state. The immune profile which must be mapped for each person tells the current situation with one's immune system. Creation of such a profile starts by performing serological analyses that offer an overview of the individual's metabolism. The process of profiling checks the patient's complete blood count, looks for blood coagulation factors, and records amounts of trace elements in the blood. German health professionals view someone's malignant tumor as the last stage in a disease process that is affecting one's entire body, and it has been manifested because of immune system breakdown.

Importance of Having a Viable Immune System

Over the past decade, extensive research has revealed how important the immune system is to the body's ability to resist acute and chronic diseases, and to function at its most effective level. Medical science now recognizes that even a healthy immune system can be affected both by our mental and emotional states and by the body's own chemical mediators such as lithium, noradrenaline, all the different cytokines, and others.

Healthy human beings are equipped with 1.5 kilograms (3.3 pounds) of a cell count totaling more than 10^{12} of immune-competent cells, which are the main component of that invisible organ, the immune system. These cells consist of a cocktail of macrophages including the white blood cells (T-lymphocytes and B-lymphocytes) which are natural killer cells, and plasma cells. Furthermore, these individual cells of the immune system are linked to each other through constant chemical feedback from within the body in response to harmful intruding organisms.

The immune system also has a countermechanism that keeps its killer and scavenger cells from destroying normal healthy tissue and organisms. This countermechanism consists of the T-suppressor cells. Suppressor cells have the power to increase the body's ability to kill incompatible organisms, and they work in conjunction with T-helper cells to balance the immune system responses. The ratio between the suppressor and helper cells determines how powerful the body's self-defense system is at any given time (in healthy people, the normal ratio is 1.2–0.3).

Dr. Helmut Keller declares, "The suppressor-helper cell ratio acts as an indicator of the body's self-defense capacity and can be used to evaluate and monitor the immune system's health."

These are the regulating mechanisms that are inherited by all humans as part of our genetic makeup. Such defense mechanisms can become diminished in persons with a history of health disorders, and even in healthy persons, the immune system can be made severely dysfunctional by chronic exposure to environmental pollutants such as smoking, too much stress, and poor diet.

Cancer Marker Tests Carried Out in Germany

Diagnosis for cancer is considered all-important by German doctors. It is aimed at recognizing a patient's physiological flaw and identifying what's required to reverse the underlying "cancer disease," which allowed the initial tumor to grow and its metastases to develop. To achieve appropriate diagnostic recognition, a comprehensive examination must be undertaken which employs many medical procedures. They involve immune function tests, dark field microscopy, blood coagulation profiling, abdominal organ ultrasound examination, heart and kidney function tests, chest X-ray and electrocardiogram, dermography-bioelectrical decoding, autonomic nervous system analysis, regulation thermography, bio-energetic testing, metabolism and digestion testing, acid-base balancing, the redox potential determination, recording the electrical resistance in blood, urine, and saliva, skin reactivity testing, general defense conditioning, and learning of overall dental health by means of panorex X-raying and testing TMJ functioning. Diagnostics prior to treatment are vital.

In contrast to cancer diagnostic practices in the United States, German oncologists such as Dr. Holger Wehner, Dr. Helmut Keller, Dr. Friedrich Douwes of the St. Georg Klinik in Bad Aibling, and others rely on numbers of cancer marker tests to determine a person's involvement with malignancy. North American oncology offers no single blood test as a valid, all-inclusive cancer marker that conclusively recognizes the presence or absence of active pathology; however, many good blood prognosticators do exist for monitoring the disease, and many of them are used in Germany.

"Immune System Biomarker Tests" on page 188 provides a series of descriptions showing biomarker tests for determining the patient's response to cancer treatment. These tests can be utilized either by themselves, in conjunction with each other, or along with additional cancer detection examinations such as biopsy, X-ray films, lymphangiography, endoscopy, cytology, radioactive scans, ultrasound, computerized tomography, and more.[1] First, however, I will provide you with full disclosure about the anti-malignin antibody in serum (AMAS) cancer marking test, which is popular among German physicians.

The AMAS Test for IgM Malignin Antibodies

Malignin is a polypeptide that often becomes part of the malignant cell's mutagenic process, something the body attempts to counter by formation of an antibody against it. This anti-malignin antibody becomes elevated in the blood sera of patients exhibiting a wide range of active malignancies regardless of the cancer site or cell type. The anti-malignin antibody or AMA shows itself, therefore, as a general transformation antibody and is not present only for one particular type of cancer. A rise early in the course of the patient's disease—as early as nineteen months before clinical detection—offers a predictive means of knowing that cancer is coming on. For blood sera determined within twenty-four hours of being drawn, the false positive and false negative rates are less than 1 percent.[2,3]

The AMAS test is a highly valuable diagnostic tool since it makes possible the recognition of cancer years earlier than possible by common laboratory tests and morphological changes. At present in conventionally practiced oncology, leading committees and institutions do not believe in the predictability of cancer. A patient must wait now until a malignant disease can be measured as morphological phenomeon; only then will health insurance companies support payment for treatment. Then the advanced stage of cancer that develops often makes such a situation too late in most cases to bring on permanent remission. *(Author's note: For further information about the AMAS test, see my published article in the June 1992 Townsend Letter for Doctors and Patients[4] or receive an article reprint by mailing a self-addressed envelope containing postage sufficient for eight ounces plus $10 to Morton Walker, D.P.M., 484 High Ridge Road, Stamford, Connecticut 06905 U.S.A.)*

Immune System Biomarker Tests

The following medical tests (some considered experimental) are utilized by German holistic oncologist Helmut Keller, M.D., to determine the immune status of his patients under treatment for cancer and/or other degenerative or infectious diseases. These are biomarkers useful for monitoring patients' responses to therapy. (See this chapter's Resource section for a U.S. laboratory source of test results.)

• AFP (alpha-fetoprotein). An enzyme immunoassay measuring protein associated with fetal tissue and malignancy. It is elevated in primary tumors of the liver and nonseminomatous testicular germ cell tumors.

• B2M (beta-2-microglobulin). A radioimmunoassay detecting the light chain of surface histocompatibility antigens on nucleated cells. B2M is the best single prognostic indicator of patient survival in multiple myeloma. The marker has utility in monitoring leukemia and lymphoma. Decreased glomerular filtration rate may elevate plasma B2M levels since this substance is cleared by the kidney.

• CA 15-3 (breast antigens 115D8/DF3). An immunoradiometric assay using monoclonal antibodies to breast carcinoma cell line MCF-7 and defatted milk fat globules. Preliminary clinical data indicate a sensitivity of 57 percent in primary preoperative breast tumors and 79 percent in metastatic breast cancer.

• CA 19-9 (carbohydrate antigen 19-9). An immunoradiometric assay using a monoclonal antibody against sialylated Lewis[a] antigen (a blood group substance) useful in pancreatic, gastric, hepatic, and recurrent colorectal carcinoma. This antigen is also termed gastrointestinal cancer–associated antigen (GICA). Patients who are Le[ab] will test negative with this assay.

• CA 125 (cancer antigen 125). An immunoradiometric assay using a monoclonal antibody (OC 125) with 88 percent sensitivity in detecting nonmucinous epithelial ovarian carcinoma and 60 percent sensitivity in detecting uterine cancer.

• CEA (carcinoembryonic antigen). An enzyme immunoassay using a monoclonal antibody against glycoprotein produced by immature and/or malignant cells originating in the gut. Elevated values are associated with carcinomas of the rectum, colon, lung, and breast.

• DM/70K (ovarian marker NB/70K). A radioimmunoassay for detecting human ovarian-tumor-associated antigen NB/70K using the monoclonal antibody NB 12123. Sensitivity of 70 percent is found in ovarian carcinoma. Elevated levels have also been associated with other gynecologic malignancies as well as carcinoma of the lung and breast.

• Ferritin. A radioimmunoassay measuring a dimeric iron-storage protein containing sialic acid. In head and neck cancers, decreasing ferritin levels are prognostic of successful therapy. In neuroblastoma, ferritin levels are used to monitor the course of the disease.

• HCG (human chorionic gonadotropin, beta sub-unit). An enzyme immunoassay measuring hormone ordinarily made by the placenta and used as an indicator of pregnancy. HCG is also produced by tumors of germ cell origin, such as testicular and ovarian as well as some lung cancers.

• IAP (immunosuppressive acidic protein). A radial immunodiffusion assay measuring a type of alpha-1-acid glycoprotein. This acidic protein suppresses phytohemagglutination-induced lymphocyte blast formation and the mixed-lymphocyte reaction in vitro. Sensitivities of 84 percent or greater are found in adenocarcinoma of the lung, pancreas, and ovary as well as leukemia and lymphoma.

• IL-2R (interleukin-2 receptor). An enzyme immunoassay for detecting soluble IL-2 receptors derived largely from activated malignant cells of lymphoproliferative or hematologic disorders (highest in hairy cell leukemia).

• LASA-P test (lipid-associated sialic acid in plasma). A biomarker, useful in a wide range of malignancies, that reflects alteration in the surface membrane of malignant cells. The LASA-P test measures total gangliosides and glycoproteins by the biochemical extraction and partition method of Dr. N. Katopodis et al. Sensitivities range from 77 percent to 97 percent depending on cell of origin of the neoplasm. Studies have shown improved predictive value when the LASA-P test is combined with other biomarkers in biomarker profiles.

Resources

For information about the anti-malignin antibody in serum (AMAS) test, contact the test's developer: Samuel Bogoch, M.D., Ph.D., chairman of the board of Oncolab, Inc., 36 The Fenway, Boston, Massachusetts 02215; telephone (800) 9CA-TEST or (800) 922-8378 or (617) 536-0850; fax (617) 535-0657. The AMAS test must be performed within twenty-four hours of blood drawing, and toward this end, Oncolab, Inc., provides the collection tubes plus the container for serum delivery.

To acquire results from the physician participation program of biomarker tests described in this chapter for investigative use only (to be used in conjunction with other medically established diagnostic procedures), contact James B. Amberson, M.D., laboratory director of Dianon Systems, 200 Watson Boulevard, Stratford, Connecticut 06497; telephone (800) 328-2666 or (203) 381-4000. The practicing physician requesting a patient's laboratory results will receive a Diagraph® Oncology Test Report with performance characteristics not yet established in conventional oncology.

APPENDIX A

Progressive Professional Health Associations

- American Association of Naturopathic Physicians. This organization provides a list of naturopaths who administer natural and nontoxic therapies; telephone (703) 556-9728; website www.naturo pathic.org.

- American Holistic Medical Association. The AHMA provides a list of holistic doctors who employ complementary and alternative medicine (CAM); telephone (703) 556-9728; website www.holis ticmedicine.org.

- American College for Advancement in Medicine. ACAM members possess the M.D., D.O., or equivalent degree with unrestricted licensure to practice medicine or engage in research in the emerging and innovative fields of holistic medical therapy and preventive medicine; telephone (949) 583-7666 or (800) 532-3688; website www.acam.org.

- The National Foundation for Alternative Medicine. The NFAM has evaluated 57 clinics in 16 countries and is developing a composite picture of how cancer patients are treated worldwide, especially throughout Europe; telephone (202) 463-4900; website www.nfam.org.

- National Center for Complementary and Alternative Medicine. This organization provides the means to find journal citations related to complementary and alternative medicine on the U.S. National Library of Medicine database; telephone (888) 644-6226; websites www.nlm.nih.gov and/or www.nccam/camonpubmed. html.

• The Natural Pharmacist. This organization provides a searchable database of vitamin, mineral, and herbal monographs describing the latest research, caveats, and cautions connected with immune-system-boosting therapies; telephone (800) 637-7784; website www.tnp.com.

APPENDIX B

Progressive American Physicians

Reprinted with permission from the American College for Advancement in Medicine (ACAM).

Author's Note: Inasmuch as this list of U.S. holistic physicians gets updated twice yearly, for the most current information you may wish to contact ACAM's director of communications, Mr. Jack Gallagher. You can reach Mr. Gallagher by phoning (800) 532-3688, extension 18, or (949) 583-7666; or fax him at (949) 455-9675; or write to the American College for Advancement in Medicine, 23121 Verdugo Drive, Suite 204, Laguna Hills, California 92653; see the ACAM website: www.acam.org.

ALABAMA
Birmingham
Michael S. Vaughn, MD
One Lakeshore Dr., #100
Birmingham, AL 35209
(205) 930-2950

Daphne
Charles Runels Jr, MD
6483 Van Buren Street
Daphne, AL 36526
(334) 625-2612 FAX (334) 625-2615

Glen P. Wilcoxson, MD
P.O. Box 1347
Daphne, AL 36526
(251) 447-0333 FAX (251) 447-0009

Fairthorpe
E. Derry Hubbard, MD
761-A Middle Avenue
Fairthorpe, AL 36532
(251) 990-0662

Gulf Shores
Gregory S. Funk, DO
2103 W. 1st Street
P.O. Box 2029
Gulf Shores, AL 36547
(251) 968-2441 FAX (251) 968-5555

Heflin
Gus J. Prosch Jr., MD
P.O. Box 427
Heflin, AL 36264
(205) 222-0960 FAX (256) 748-3126

Montgomery
Teresa D. Allen, DO
6715 Taylor Court
Montgomery, AL 36117
(334) 273-0904 FAX (334) 273-0905

Scott Bell, MD
7020 Sydney Curve
Montgomery, AL 36117
(334) 277-5363 FAX (334) 277-5362

ALASKA
Anchorage
Sandra Denton, MD
3333 Denali Street #100
Alaska Alternative Medicine
Clinic, LLC
Anchorage, AK 99503
(907) 563-6200 FAX (907) 561-7933

Robert Thompson, MD
3333 Denali Street, #100
Anchorage, AK 99503
(907) 563-6200 FAX (907) 561-4933

Kenai
Elisabeth-Anne Cole, MD
11568 Kenai Spur Hwy., #1
Kenai, AK 99611
(907) 283-7740 FAX (907) 283-7760

Kodiak
Ronald Brockman, DO
P.O. Box 95
Kodiak, AK 99615
(907) 563-9166 FAX (907) 563-9466

ARIZONA
Cave Creek
Frank W. George, DO
6748 E. Lone Mountain Rd.
Cave Creek, AZ 85331
(480) 595-5508 FAX (480) 575-1570

Flagstaff
Marnie Vail, MD
702 North Beaver Street
Flagstaff, AZ 86001
(928) 214-9774 FAX (928) 214-9772

Glendale
Lloyd D. Armold, DO
7200 W. Bell Rd., #G-103
Glendale, AZ 85308
(623) 939-8916 FAX (623) 978-2817

Mesa
Thomas J. Grade, MD
6309 E. Baywood Ave.
Mesa, AZ 85206
(480) 325-3801 FAX (480) 981-1309

Charles D. Schwengel, DO
1050 E. University Drive, #4
Mesa, AZ 85203
(602) 668-1448

Paradise Valley
Alan K. Ketover, MD
10595 N. Tatum Blvd., #E-146
Paradise Valley, AZ 85253
(602) 381-0800 FAX (602) 381-0054

Parker
Jeff A. Baird, DO
1413 - 16th Street
Parker, AZ 85344
(928) 669-9229

Payson
Garry F. Gordon, MD
708 E. Hwy., 260, Bldg. C-1, #F
Payson, AZ 85541
(928) 472-4263 FAX (928) 474-3819

Phoenix
Edward C. Kondrot, MD
2001 W. Camelback Rd., #150
Phoenix, AZ 85015
(602) 347-7950

Scottsdale
Gordon H. Josephs, DO
7315 E. Evans Road
Scottsdale, AZ 85260
(480) 998-9232 - FAX (480) 998-1528

Sedona
Lester Adler, MD
40 Soldiers Pass Rd., #12

Sedona, AZ 86336
(520) 282-2520

Mark E. Laursen, MD
150 Thunderbird Drive
Sedona, AZ 86336
(520) 204-0023 FAX (520) 204-1571

Annemarie S. Welch, MD
2301 West Hwy. 89A, #104
Sedona, AZ 86336
(928) 282-0609 FAX (928) 282-9401

ARKANSAS
Little Rock
Norbert J. Becquet, MD
613 Main Street
Little Rock, AR 72201
(501) 375-4419 FAX (501) 375-4067

Springdale
Jeffrey R. Baker, MD
900 Dorman St., #E
Springdale, AR 72762
(479) 756-3251

CALIFORNIA
Atascadero
Carmelo A. Plateroti, DO
Dermatology
8548 El Camino Real
Atascadero, CA 93422
(805) 462-2262 FAX (805) 462-2264

Azusa
William C. Bryce, MD, DO, PhD
400 N. San Gabriel Ave.
Azusa, CA 91702-3446
(626) 334-1407 FAX (626) 334-1116

Bakersfield
Shivinder Deol, MD
4000 Stockdale Hwy. #D
Bakersfield, CA 93309
(661) 325-7452 FAX (661) 325-7456

Beverly Hills
Cathie Ann Lippman, MD
291 S. La Cienega Bl., Suite 207

Beverly Hills, CA 90211
(310) 289-8430

Burbank
David J. Edwards, MD
2202 W. Magnolia
Burbank, CA 91506
(818) 842-4184 (800) 975-2202

Douglas Hunt, MD
3808 Riverside Dr., #510
Burbank, CA 91505
(818) 566-9889 FAX (818) 566-9879

Nancy T. Mullan, MD
2829 West Burbank Blvd., #202
Burbank, CA 91505
(818) 954-9267 FAX (818) 954-0620

Burney
Charles K. Dahlgren, MD
37491 Enterprise Dr., #C
Burney, CA 96013
(530) 335-3833

Carmel
Jerry A. Wyker, MD
25530 Rio Vista Drive
Carmel, CA 93923
(831) 625-0911 FAX (831) 625-0467

Carmel Valley
Howard Press, MD
13748 Center St., #B
Carmel Valley, CA 93924
(831) 659-5373 FAX (831) 659-5290

Carmichael
Bernard McGinity, MD
6945 Fair Oaks Blvd.
Carmichael, CA 95608
(916) 485-4556 FAX (916) 485-1491

Philip J. Reilly, MD
4800 Manzanita Ave., #17
Carmichael, CA 95608
(916) 488-9524

Chula Vista
Luis Perez, MD
790 Otay Lakes Rd.

Chula Vista, CA 91910
(619) 216-1600 FAX (619) 216-1616

Concord
John Toth, MD
2299 Bacon St., #10
Concord, CA 94520
(925) 687-9447 FAX (925) 687-9483

John Toth, Jr., DO
2299 Bacon St., #10
Concord, CA 94520
(925) 687-9447 FAX (925) 687-9483

Covina
James Privitera, MD
256 W. San Bernadino Ave.
Covina, CA 91723
(626) 966-1618 FAX (626) 966-7226

Diamond Bar
Hitendra Shah, MD
23341 Golden Springs Dr., #208
Diamond Bar, CA 91765
(909) 860-2610 FAX (909) 860-1192

Duarte
Paddy Jim Baggot, MD
931 N. Buena Vista #301
Duarte, CA 91010
(626) 358-8045 (626) 358-8216

El Cajon
Neil W. Hirschenbein, MD, PhD
1685 E. Main St., #301
El Cajon, CA 92021
(619) 579-8681 FAX (619) 579-0759

David A. Howe, MD
505 N. Mollison Ave., #103
El Cajon, CA 92021
(619) 440-3838 FAX (760) 489-2238

William J. Saccoman, MD
505 N. Mollison Ave., Suite 103
El Cajon, CA 92021
(619) 440-3838 FAX (619) 440-8293

Encinitas
Mark Drucker, MD
4403 Manchester Ave., #107

Encinitas, CA 92024
(760) 632-9042 FAX (760) 632-0574

Encino
Ilona Abraham, MD
17815 Ventura Blvd., Stes. 111 & 113
Encino, CA 91316
(818) 345-8721 FAX (818) 345-7150

Escondido
Aline Fournier, DO
307 S. Ivy
Escondido, CA 92025
(760) 746-1133 FAX (760) 746-9880

Ratibor Pantovich, DO
560 E. Valley Pkwy.
Escondido, CA 92025
(760) 480-2880 FAX (760) 480-0102

Fountain Valley
Allen Green, MD
18153 Brookhurst St.
Fountain Valley, CA 92708
(714) 378-5656 FAX (714) 378-5650

Fresno
David J. Edwards, MD
360 S. Clovis Ave.
Fresno, CA 93727
(559) 251-5066 FAX (559) 251-5108

Patrick A. Golden, MD
1187 E. Herndon, #101
Fresno, CA 93720
(559) 432-0716 FAX (559) 432-4545

Glendale
Abraham Maissian, MD
1737 W. Glenoaks Blvd.
Glendale, CA 91201
(818) 243-1186 FAX (818) 243-3868

Hemet
Hitendra Shah, MD
229 West 7th
Hemet, CA 92583
(909) 487-2550 FAX (909) 487-2552

Huntington Beach
Francis Foo, MD
10188 Adams Ave.
Huntington Beach, CA 92646
(714) 968-3266 FAX (714) 968-6408

Indio
Robert Harmon, MD
41-800 Washington St., #110
Indio, CA 92201-8154
(619) 345-2696

Irvine
Allan E. Sosin, MD
16100 Sand Canyon Ave., #240
Irvine, CA 92618
(949) 753-8889 FAX (949) 753-0410

Ronald Wempen, MD
14795 Jeffrey Rd., Suite 101
Irvine, CA 92618
(949) 551-8751 FAX (949) 551-1272

La Jolla
Charles Moss, MD
8950 Villa La Jolla, #2162
La Jolla, CA 92037
(619) 457-1314 FAX (619) 457-3615

Laguna Hills
Peter Muran, MD
23521 Paseo de Valencia, #204
Laguna Hills, CA 92653
(949) 472-3717 FAX (714) 430-1443

Laguna Niguel
Tori Danielle, MD
24 Bethany
Laguna Niguel, CA 92677

Lake Forest
Michael Grossman, MD
24432 Muirlands Blvd., #111
Lake Forest, CA 92630
(949) 770-7301 FAX (949) 770-0634

Lancaster
Richard P. Huemer, MD
1739 West Avenue J

Lancaster, CA 93534
(661) 945-4502 FAX (661) 945-4841

Long Beach
H. R. Casdorph, MD
1703 Termino Ave., Suite 201
Long Beach, CA 90804
(562) 597-8716 FAX (562) 597-4616

Los Altos
Robert F. Cathcart III, MD
127 Second St., Suite 4
Los Altos, CA 94022
(650) 949-2822

F. T. Guilford, MD
5050 El Camino Real, #110
Los Altos, CA 94022
(650) 964-6700 FAX (650) 433-0947

Raj Patel, MD
5050 El Camino Real, #110
Los Altos, CA 94022
(650) 964-6700 FAX (650) 964-3495

D. Graeme Shaw, MD
5050 El Camino Real, #110
Los Altos, CA 94022
(650) 964-6700 FAX (650) 964-3495

Los Angeles
Michael Galitzer, MD
12381 Wilshire Blvd., #102
Los Angeles, CA 90025
(310) 820-6042 FAX (310) 207-3342

Hans D. Gruenn, MD
2211 Corinth Ave., #204
Los Angeles, CA 90064
(310) 966-9194 FAX (310) 966-9196

Karima Hirani, MD
12732-B W. Washington Blvd.
Los Angeles, CA 90066
(310) 577-0753 FAX (310) 577-0728

Charles Law Jr., MD
3400 Ben Lomond Place, #304
Los Angeles, CA 90027-2956
(818) 761-1661

Murray Susser, MD
2211 Corinth Ave., #204

Los Angeles, CA 90064
(310) 966-9194 FAX (310) 966-9196

Los Gatos
Phillip Lee Miller, MD
15215 National Ave., #103
Los Gatos, CA 95032
(408) 358-8855

Mission Hills
Sion Nobel, MD
10306 N. Sepulveda Blvd.
Mission Hills, CA 91345
(818) 361-0115 FAX (818) 361-9497

Modesto
Christine G. Tazewell, MD
1524 McHenry Ave., #310
Modesto, CA 95350-4570
(209) 575-4700 FAX (209) 577-6699

Monterey
Denise Mark, MD
Monterey Bay Wellness
659 Abrego St., #6
Monterey, CA 93940
(831) 642-9266 FAX (831) 642-9276

Napa
Eleanor Hynote, MD
935 Trancas Street, Ste. 1A
Napa, CA 94558
(707) 255-4172 FAX (707) 255-2605

Newport Beach
Catherine Arvantely, MD
4321 Birch Street, #100
Newport Beach, CA 92660
(949) 851-1550 FAX (949) 955-3005

Julian Whitaker, MD
4321 Birch St., Suite 100
Newport Beach, CA 92660
(949) 851-1550 FAX (949) 955-3005

North Hollywood
Christine Daniel, MD
12650 Sherman Way, #4
N. Hollywood, CA 91605
(818) 982-8062 FAX (818) 982-8794

Oceanside
Ratibor Pantovich, DO
1002 South Coast Hwy.
Oceanside, CA 92054
(760) 439-9933 FAX (760) 439-3463

Palm Desert
Robert Neal Rouzier, MD
77564B Country Club Dr., #320
Palm Desert, CA 92211
(760) 772-8883

Palm Springs
David Freeman, MD
2825 Tahquitz Canyon, #200
Palm Springs, CA 92262
(760) 320-4292

Robert Neal Rouzier, MD
2825 Tahquitz Canyon, Suite 200
Palm Springs, CA 92262
(760) 320-4292 (760) 322-9475

Priscilla A. Slagle, MD
946 Avenida Palos Verdes
Palm Springs, CA 92262
(760) 323-4259 FAX (760) 323-4259

Redding
Bessie J. Tillman, MD
2787 Eureka Way, Suite 1-1
Redding, CA 96001
(530) 246-3022 FAX (530) 246-7894

Redlands
Felix Prakasam, MD
2048 Orange Tree Lane
Redlands, CA 92374
(909) 798-1614

Sacramento
Michael Kwiker, DO
3301 Alta Arden, Suite 3
Sacramento, CA 95825
(916) 489-4400 FAX (916) 489-1710

San Diego
Neal W. Hirschenbein, MD, PhD
9339 Genesee Ave., #150
San Diego, CA 92122
(858) 713-9401

Michael Leeman, MD
8950 Villa La Jolla Dr., #A-126
San Diego, CA 92037
(858) 550-1999 FAX (858-550-1955

Romeo A. Quini, MD
7808 Clairemont Mesa Blvd., #D
San Diego, CA 92111
(858) 565-0060 FAX (760) 839-0298

San Francisco
Paul Lynn, MD
345 W. Portal Ave., 2nd Floor
San Francisco, CA 94127
(415) 566-1000 FAX (415) 665-6732

Wai-Man Ma, MD
728 Pacific Ave., #611
San Francisco, CA 94133
(415) 397-3888

Gary Ross, MD
500 Sutter, #300
San Francisco, CA 94102
(415) 398-0555 FAX (415) 398-6228

San Jose
Carl L. Ebnother, MD
7174 Santa Teresa Blvd., #6-A
San Jose, CA 95139
(408) 363-1498

San Ramon
Richard Gracer, MD
5401 Norris Canyon Rd., #102
San Ramon, CA 94583
(925) 277-1100 FAX (925) 283-2009

Santa Barbara
Kenneth J. Frank, MD
831 State St., #280
Santa Barbara, CA 93101
(805) 730-7420 FAX (805) 730-7434

James L. Kwako, MD
1805-D East Cabrillo Blvd.
Santa Barbara, CA 93018
(805) 565-3959 FAX (805) 565-3989

Bob Young, MD
119 North Milpas

Santa Barbara, CA 93103
(805) 963-1824 FAX (805) 963-1826

Santa Monica
Joseph Sciabbarrasi, MD
1821 Wilshire Blvd., #400
Santa Monica, CA 90403
(310) 828-4175 FAX (310) 828-4324

Santa Rosa
Ron Kennedy, MD
2448 Guerneville Rd., Ste. 800
Santa Rosa, CA 95403
(707) 576-0100

Sebastopol
Isaac Eliaz, MD
721 Jonive Rd.
Sebastopol, CA 95472
(707) 829-5900 FAX (707) 874-1815

Norman Zucker, MD
867 Gravenstein Hwy. South
Sebastopol, CA 95472-4522
(707) 823-6116 or (800) 799-2250

Stanton
William J. Goldwag, MD
7499 Cerritos Ave.
Stanton, CA 90680
(714) 827-5180

Templeton
Carmelo A. Plateroti, DO
1111 Las Tablas Rd.,#M
Templeton, CA 93465
(805) 434-2821 FAX (805) 434-2526

Tustin
Leigh Erin Connealy, MD
14642 Newport Ave., #200
Tustin, CA 92780
(714) 669-4446 FAX (714) 669-4448

Allan Harvey Lane, MD
12581 Newport Avenue, Ste. B
Tustin, CA 92780
(714) 544-9544 FAX (714) 544-9611

Ukiah
Lawrence G. Foster, MD
230 B Hospital Drive
Ukiah, CA 95482
(707) 463-3502

Upland
Bryan P. Chan, MD
1148 San Bernardino Rd., #E-102
Upland, CA 91786
(909) 920-3578 FAX (909) 949-1238

Vista
Les Breitman, MD
Institute for Anti-Aging Medicine
2023 W. Vista Way, Ste. F
Vista, CA 92083
(760) 414-9955 FAX (760) 414-9933

West Toluca Lake
Salvacion Lee, MD
11336 Camarillo St., #305
West Toluca Lake, CA 91602
(818) 505-1574 FAX (818) 505-1574

COLORADO
Aurora
Terry A. Grossman, MD
3150 S. Peoria St., Unit H
Aurora, CO 80014
(303) 338-1323 FAX (303) 338-1324

Boulder
Michael A. Zeligs, MD
1000 Alpine, #211
Boulder, CO 80304
(303) 442-5492 FAX (303) 447-3610

Broomfield
Ron Rosedale, MD
P O Box 6278
Broomfield, CO 80030
(303) 530-5555 FAX (303) 530-5522

Colorado Springs
George Juetersonke, DO
3525 American Drive
Colorado Springs, CO 80917
(719) 597-6075 FAX (719) 573-6529

Joel Klein, MD
5455 N. Union Blvd.,#201
Colorado Springs, CO 80918
(719) 457-0330 FAX (719) 457-0860

Denver
Terry Grossman, MD
2801 Youngfield
Denver, CO 80401
(303) 233-4247 FAX (303) 233-4249

Durango
Ronald E. Wheeler, MD
2901 Main Avenue
Durango, CO 81301
(970) 259-4081 FAX (970) 247-3074

Fort Collins
Roger Billica, MD
1020 Luke Street, #A
Fort Collins, CO 80524
(970) 495-0999 FAX (970) 495-1016

Grand Junction
Joseph M. Wezensky, MD
2650 North Ave., Suite 101
Grand Junction, CO 81501
(970) 263-4660 FAX (970) 248-9519

Greenwood Village
Susanna S. Choi, MD
8200 E. Belleview Ave., #240E
Greenwood Village, CO 80111
(303) 721-1670 FAX (303) 721-8117

Lakewood
Terry A. Grossman, MD
2801 Youngfield St., #117
Lakewood, CO 80401
(303) 233-4247 FAX (303) 233-4249

Snowmass
Rob Krakovitz, MD
0094 Elk Ridge Drive
Snowmass, CO 81654
(970) 927-4394

CONNECTICUT
Bridgeport
Tadeusz A. Skowron, MD
50 Ridgefield Ave., #317
Bridgeport, CT 06610
(203) 368-1450

Hamden
Robert Lang, MD
60 Washington Ave., #105
Hamden, CT 06518-3272
(203) 248-4362 FAX (203) 248-6933

Madison
Robert Lang, MD
11 Woodland Road
Madison, CT 06443
(203) 318-5264

Milford
Alan R. Cohen, MD
67 Cherry Street
Milford, CT 06460
(203) 877-1936

Ridgefield
Marcie Wolinsky-Friedland, MD
31 Bayley Avenue
Americas Medical Center
Ridgefield, CT 06877
(203) 431-6165 FAX (203) 431-6167

Stamford
Henry C. Sobo, MD
122 Hoyt St., #D
Stamford, CT 06905
(203) 348-8805 FAX (203) 348-6398

Torrington
Jerrold N. Finnie, MD
333 Kennedy Dr., #204
Torrington, CT 06790
(860) 489-8977

Wilton
Warren Levin, MD
13 Powder Horn Hill
Wilton, CT 06897-3122
(203) 834-1174 FAX (203) 834-1175

DELAWARE
New Castle
Jeffrey K. Kerner, DO
200 Bassett Ave.
New Castle, DE 19720
(302) 328-0669 FAX (302) 328-8937

DIST. OF COLUMBIA
Washington
George H. Mitchell, MD
2639 Connecticut Ave. NW,
Suite C-100
Washington, DC 20008
(202) 265-4111

Bruce Rind, MD
5225 Wisconsin Ave., NW
4th Floor
Washington, DC 20015
(202) 237-7000

Aldo M. Rosemblat, MD
5225 Wisconsin Ave. N.W., #401
Washington, DC 20015
(202) 237-7000 FAX (202) 237-0017

FLORIDA
Apopka
Allan Zubkin, MD
424 N. Park Ave.
Apopka, FL 32712
(407) 886-0611 FAX (407) 886-2817

Beverly Hills
James Lemire, MD
4065 N. Lecanto Hwy., #100
Beverly Hills, FL 34465
(352) 527-6840 FAX (352) 527-6843

Boca Raton
Leonard Haimes, MD
7300 N. Federal Hwy.,# 100
Boca Raton, FL 33487-1631
(561) 995-8484 FAX (561) 995-7773

Bonita Springs
Stephen Kaskie, MD
#2100 - 3501 Health Center Blvd.
Bonita Springs, FL 39135
(941) 948-2000 FAX (941) 948-2058

Dean R. Silver, MD
9240 Bonita Beach Rd., #2215
Gulfcoast Longevity and Wellness
Center
Bonita Springs, FL 34135
(941) 949-0101 FAX (941) 949-4334

Boynton Beach
Kenneth Lee, MD
1501 Corporate Dr., #240
Boynton Beach, FL 33426
(561) 736-8806

Bradenton
Eteri Melnikov, MD
116 Manatee Ave. East
Bradenton, FL 34208
(941) 748-7943 FAX (941) 748-1258

Clearwater
Donald J. Carrow, MD
4908 Creekside Dr., #A
Clearwater, FL 34620
(727) 573-3775 FAX (727) 556-0082

David Minkoff, MD
301 Turner Street
Clearwater, FL 33756
(727) 442-5612

David M. Wall, MD
1749 Long Bow Lane
Clearwater, FL 33764
(727) 724-0135 FAX (727) 724-0129

Coral Springs
Jerald H. Ratner, MD
9750 N.W. 33rd St., #211
Coral Springs, FL 33065
(954) 752-9450 FAX (954) 752-9888

Anthony J. Sancetta, DO
8217 W. Atlantic Blvd.
Coral Springs, FL 33071
(954) 757-1211 FAX (954) 757-1255

Daytona Beach
John Ortolani, MD
1430 Mason Ave.
Daytona Beach, FL 32117
(386) 274-3601 FAX (386) 274-2009

Fort Lauderdale
Cristino C. Enriquez, MD
767 S. State Road 7
Fort Lauderdale, FL 33317
(954) 583-3335 FAX (954) 463-8006

Bach A. McComb, DO, ND, PhD
1655 E. Oakland Park Blvd
Fort Lauderdale, FL 33334
(954) 661-2225

Fort Myers
Robert A. Didonato, MD
3443 Hancock Bridge Pkwy., #301
N. Ft. Myers, FL 33903
(941) 997-8800 FAX (941) 997-7706

Gary L. Pynckel, DO
3840 Colonial Blvd., #1
Fort Myers, FL 33912
(941) 278-3377 FAX (941) 278-3702

Gainesville
Robert Erickson, MD
905 NW 56th Terrace, Ste. B
Gainesville, FL 32605
(352) 331-5138 FAX (352) 331-9399

Hanoch Talmor, MD
4421 NW 39th Ave., Bldg. 2-1
Gainesville, FL 32606-7214
(352) 377-0015 FAX (352) 378-1895

Hialeah
Francisco Mora, MD
1490 West 48th Place, #398
Hialeah, FL 33012
(305) 820-6211 FAX (305) 822-0116

Hollywood
Michelle Morrow, DO
5821 Hollywood Blvd.
Hollywood, FL 33021
(954) 436-6363 FAX (954) 436-6731

Homosassa Springs
Carlos F. Gonzalez, MD
7989 So. Suncoast Blvd.
Homosassa Springs, FL 32646
(352) 382-2900 FAX (352) 382-1633

Indialantic
Glen Wagner, MD
121 - 6th Ave.
Indialantic, FL 32903
(407) 723-5915

Indian Harbour Beach
Daniel B. Hammond, MD
1413 South Patrick Drive
Indian Harbour Beach, FL 32937
(407) 777-9923 FAX (407) 777-4707

Jacksonville
Norman S. Cohen, MD
5150 Belfort Road, Bldg. 400
The Vein Clinic & Longevity
Center
Jacksonville, FL 32256-6026
(904) 296-0900 FAX (904) 296-8346

Stephen Grable, MD
7563 Philips Hwy., #206
Jacksonville, FL 32256
(904) 824-8353 FAX (904)296-1472

Key Biscayne
Sam Baxas, MD
30 West Mashta Drive, Ste. 200
Key Biscayne, FL 33149
(305) 361-9249 FAX (305) 361-2179

Kissimmee
Carmelita Bamba-Dagani, MD
500 North John Young Pkwy.
Kissimmee, FL 34741
(407) 935-1060 FAX (407) 931-2056

Lady Lake
Nelson Kraucak, MD
Suite 1702
1501 US Highway 441 No.
Lady Lake, FL 32159
(352) 750-4333 FAX (352) 750-2023

Lake City
Barnie Vanzant, MD
503 S. Hernando St.
Lake City, FL 32025
(904) 752-9222

Lake Mary
Diab Ashrap, MD
3859 Lake Emma Rd.
Lake Mary, FL 32746
(407) 805-9222 FAX (407) 444-5299

Jeffrey Mueller, MD
635 Primera Blvd., #111
Lake Mary, FL 32746
(407) 833-3881 FAX (407) 833-3883

Lake Worth
Sherri W. Pinsley, DO
2290 - 10th Ave. North, #605
Lake Worth, FL 33461
(561) 547-2770

Lakeland
Harold Robinson, MD
4406 S. Florida Ave., Suite 27
Lakeland, FL 33803
(941) 646-5088

S. Todd Robinson, MD
4406 S. Florida Ave., Suite 30
Lakeland, FL 33803
(941) 646-5088

Lauderhill
Herbert R. Slavin, MD
7200 W. Commercial Blvd.,
Suite #210
Lauderhill, FL 33319
(954) 748-4991 FAX (954) 748-5022

Lecanto
Azael P. Borromeo, MD
2653 N. Lecanto Hwy.
Lecanto, FL 34461
(352) 527-9555 FAX (352) 527-2609

Longwood
Donald E. Colbert, MD
1908 Booth Circle
Longwood, FL 32750
(407) 331-7007 FAX (407) 331-5777

Marco Island
Richard Saitta, MD
1010 N. Barfield Dr.

Marco Island, FL 34145
(941) 642-8488

Melbourne
Neil Ahner, MD
1270 N. Wickham Road
Melbourne, FL 32935
(321) 253-2009 FAX (321) 253-5561

Rajiv Chandra, MD
20 E. Melbourne Ave., #104
Melbourne, FL 32901
(407) 951-7404

Glenn R. Johnston, MD
6300 N. Wickham Rd.
Melbourne, FL 32940
(321) 253-2169 FAX (321) 253-1720

Miami
Joseph G. Godorov, DO
9055 S.W. 87th Ave., Suite 307
Miami, FL 33176
(305) 595-0671

Ivonne F. Torre-Coya, MD
10534 S.W. 8th
Miami, FL 33174
(305) 223-0132 FAX (305) 553-6488

Miami Beach
Roy Heilbron, MD
6302 Alton Rd., #530
Miami Beach, FL 33140
(305) 531-6886 FAX (305) 532-9992

Miami Springs
Angelique Hart, MD
1 South Drive
Miami Springs, FL 33166
(305) 882-1442 FAX (305) 889-1040

Milton
William Watson, MD
5536 Stewart Street
Milton, FL 32570
(850) 623-3836 FAX (850) 623-2201

Mount Dora
Jack E. Young, MD, PhD
2260 W. Old US Hwy. 441

Mount Dora, FL 32757
(352) 385-4400 FAX (352) 385-4402

N. Miami Beach
Stefano DiMauro, MD
16695 N.E. 10th Avenue
N. Miami Beach, FL 33162
(305) 940-6474 FAX (305) 944-8601

Wynne A. Steinsnyder, DO
17291 N.E. 19th Avenue
N. Miami Beach, FL 33162
(305) 947-0618 FAX (305) 940-1345

Naples
David Perlmutter, MD
800 Goodlette Rd. N., #270
Naples, FL 33940
(239) 649-7400 FAX (239) 649-6370

New Smyrna Beach
William Campbell Douglass, III, MD
2111 Ocean Drive
New Smyrna Beach, FL 32169
(386) 426-8803 FAX (509) 421-8604

Ocala
George Graves, DO
11512 County Road 316
P. O. Box 2220
Ocala (Ft. McCoy), FL 32134-2220
(352) 236-2525 FAX (352) 236-8610

Orange City
Travis L. Herring, MD
106 West Fern Dr.
Orange City, FL 32763
(386) 775-0525 FAX (386) 775-3911

Orlando
Kirti Kalidas, MD
6651 Vineland Road, #150
Orlando, FL 32819
(407) 355-9246 FAX (407) 370-4774

Robert J. Rogers, MD
2170 West State Road 434, #190
Orlando, FL 32779
(407) 682-5222 FAX (407) 682-5274

Ormond Beach
Hana Chaim, DO
595 W. Granada Blvd., #D
Ormond Beach, FL 32174
(386) 672-9000

Palm Beach Gardens
Neil Ahner, MD
10333 N. Military Trail, Ste. A
Palm Beach Gardens, FL 33410
(561) 630-3696 FAX (561) 630-1991

Carlos M. Garcia, MD
36555 U.S. Hwy. 19 North
Palm Harbor, FL 34684
(727) 771-9669 FAX (727) 771-8071

Panama City
Naima Abdel-Ghany, MD, PhD
PM, Anti-Aging Med.
2424 B Frankford Avenue
Panama City, FL 32405
(850) 872-8122 FAX (850) 872-9925

James W. De Ruiter, MD
2202 State Ave., #311
Panama City, FL 32405
(850) 747-4963 FAX (850) 747-0074

Samir M.A. Yassin, MD
516 S. Tyndall Pkwy., #202
Panama City, FL 32404
(850) 763-0464

Pensacola
Lucey R.W., MD
Madison Office Park
4300 Bayou Blvd., #27
Pensacola, FL 32503
(850) 477-3453 FAX (850) 474-9420

Plantation
Adam Frent, DO
1741 N. University Drive
Plantation, FL 33322
(954) 474-1617 FAX (954) 472-1631

Alvin Stein, MD
4101 NW 4 St., #S-401
Plantation, FL 33317
(954) 581-8585 FAX (954) 581-5580

Punta Gorda
James Coy, MD
310 Nesbit St., P.O. Box 511315
Punta Gorda, FL 33951
(941) 575-8080 FAX (941) 575-8108

Sarasota
W. Frederic Harvey, MD
3982 Bee Ridge Rd., Bldg.H, #J
Sarasota, FL 34239
(941) 929-9355

Rebecca Roberts, DO
1521 Dolphin St., #10
Sarasota, FL 34236
(941) 365-6273 FAX (941) 365-4269

Alan Sault, MD
2000 So. Tamiami Trail
Sarasota, FL 34239
(941) 955-5579

Ronald E. Wheeler, MD
The Sarasota City Center
1819 Main St., Ste. 401
Sarasota, FL 34236
(941) 957-0007

Sebastian
Peter Holyk, MD
600 Schumann Drive
Sebastian, FL 32958
(772) 338-5554 FAX (772) 388-2410

Spring Hill
Nabil Habib, MD
3300 Josef Avenue
Spring Hill, FL 34609
(352) 683-1166 FAX (352) 683-2902

Calin V. Pop, MD
4215 Rachel Boulevard
Spring Hill, FL 34607
(352) 597-2240 FAX (352) 597-2990

St. Petersburg
John P. Lenhart, MD
6110 - 9th Street N.
St. Petersburg, FL 33703
(727) 526-0600 FAX (727) 345-0928

Ray Wunderlich Jr., MD
1152 - 94th Ave. North
St. Petersburg, FL 33702
(727) 822-3612 FAX (727) 578-1370

Stuart
Neil Ahner, MD
705 North Federal Hwy.
Stuart, FL 34994
(561) 692-9200 FAX (561) 692-9888

Sherri W. Pinsley, DO
7000 S.E. Federal Hwy., Suite #302
Stuart, FL 34997
(561) 220-1697 FAX (561) 220-7332

Sunny Isles Beach
Martin Dayton, DO
18600 Collins Ave.
Sunny Isles Beach, FL 33160
(305) 931-8484 FAX (305) 936-1849

Tallahassee
William Watson, MD
1630-A North Plaza Drive
Tallahassee, FL 32308
(850) 878-2888

Tamarac
George A. Lustig, MD
7401 N. University Dr., #101
Tamarac, FL 33321
(954) 724-0099 FAX (954) 724-0070

Tampa
Jean M. Allen, DO
4212 S. Manhattan Avenue
Tampa, FL 33611
(813) 837-8591

Robert J. Casanas, MD
4810 Bay Heron Place, #1012
Tampa, FL 33661
(813) 390-3037

Carlos M. Garcia, MD
4710 Havana Ave., #107
Tampa, FL 33616
(813) 350-0140 FAX (813) 350-0713

Eugene H. Lee, MD
1804 W. Kennedy Blvd. #A
Tampa, FL 33606
(813) 251-3089 FAX (813) 251-5668

Tavares
Nelson Kraucak, MD
204 N. Texas Avenue
Tavares, FL 32778
(352) 742-1116 FAX (352) 742-8288

Umatilla
Louis Radnothy, DO
390 S. Central, P.O. Drawer 2325
Umatilla, FL 32784
(352) 669-3175 FAX (352) 669-3640

Venice
Matthew Burks, MD
420 Nokomis Ave., So.
Venice, FL 34285
(941) 488-8112 FAX (941) 488-7442

Arlene Martone, MD
4140 Woodmere Park Blvd., #2
Venice, FL 34293
(941) 408-9838

Vero Beach
Neil Ahner, MD
717 17th Street
Vero Beach, FL 32960
(561) 978-0057 FAX (561) 978-9652

John Song, MD
1360 U.S. 1, #1
Vero Beach, FL 32960
(561) 770-2070 FAX (561) 569-1593

West Palm Beach
Daniel N. Tucker, MD
1411 N. Flagler Dr., #6700
West Palm Beach, FL 33401
(561) 835-0055 FAX (561) 835-1742

Winter Park
Joya Lynn Schoen, MD
1850 Lee Road, Ste. 240
Winter Park, FL 32789
(407) 644-2729 FAX (407) 644-1205

GEORGIA

Alpharetta
James Bean, MD
9690 Vantana Way, Ste. A
Alpharetta, GA 30022
(770) 418-1800

Atlanta
M. Truett Bridges, Jr, MD
4920 Roswell Rd., #35
Atlanta, GA 30342
(404) 843-8880 FAX (404) 843-8687

Stephen B. Edelson, MD
3833 Roswell Rd., #110
Atlanta, GA 30342
(404) 841-0088 FAX (404) 841-6416

Milton Fried, MD
4426 Tilly Mill Road
Atlanta, GA 30360
(770) 451-4857 FAX (770) 451-8492

Susan E. Kolb, MD
4370 Georgetown Square
Atlanta, GA 30338
(770) 390-0012 FAX (770) 457-4428

William Richardson, MD
3280 Howell Mill Rd., #205
Atlanta, GA 30327
(404) 350-9607 FAX (404) 350-9481

Brunswick
Ralph G. Ellis Jr, MD
158 Scranton Connector
Brunswick, GA 31525
(912) 280-0304 FAX (912) 280-0601

Canton
William Early, MD
320 Hospital Rd.
Canton, GA 30114
(770) 479-5535 FAX (770) 720-3294

Cartersville
Claude R. Poliak, MD
17 Bowens Court SE
Cartersville, GA 30120
(770) 607-0220 FAX (770) 607-0208

Columbus
Jan McBarron, MD
2904 Macon Rd.
Columbus, GA 31906
(706) 322-4073 FAX (706) 323-4786

Fort Oglethorpe
Charles C. Adams, MD
100 Thomas Rd.
Fort Oglethorpe, GA 30742-3617
(706) 861-7377 FAX (706) 861-7922

Gainesville
John L. Givogre, MD
530 Springs Street
Gainesville, GA 30501
(770) 503-7222

Kathryn Herndon, MD
530 Spring St.
Gainesville, GA 30503
(770) 503-7222

Macon
James T. Alley, MD
2518 Riverside Dr.
Macon, GA 31204
(478) 745-3727 or (800) 547-9743

Marietta
Ralph Lee, MD
110 Lewis Dr., Ste. B
Marietta, GA 30060
(770) 423-0064 FAX (770) 423-9827

Oglethorpe
Elwin Glynn Taunton, DO
100 Riverview Lane
P.O. Box 1069
Oglethorpe, GA 31068
(912) 472-2550 (912) 472-2555

Roswell
Marcia V. Byrd, MD
11050 Crabapple Rd., #105-B
Roswell, GA 30075
(770) 587-1711

Savannah
Yusuf Saleeby, MD

144 Habersham St.
Savannah, GA 31401
(912) 201-9464 FAX (912) 201-9467

Smyrna
Donald Ruesink, MD
1004 Lincoln Trace Cir. SE
Smyrna, GA 30080
(770) 818-9908

Stockbridge
Michael Rowland, MD
130 Eagle Springs Court, Ste. A
Stockbridge, GA 30281
(770) 507-2930 FAX (770) 507-0837

T.R. Shantha, MD, PhD
115 Eagle Spring Dr.
Stockbridge, GA 30281
(770) 474-4029 FAX (770) 474-2038

Wetumpka
Mark Hayden, MD
776297 Tallahassee Hwy.
Wetumpka, GA 36092
(334) 514-1910 FAX (334) 567-3025

HAWAII
Honolulu
Frederick Lam, MD
1270 Queen Emma St., #501
Honolulu, HI 96813
(808) 537-3311 FAX (808) 946-0378

Pritam Tapryal, MD
1270 Queen Emma St. #501
Honolulu, HI 96813
(808) 537-3311 FAX (808) 536-6361

Kapaa, Kauai
Thomas R. Yarema, MD
4504 Kukui St., #13
Kapaa, Kauai, HI 96741
(808) 823-0994 FAX (808) 823-0995

Kealakekua
Cliff Arrington, MD
P.O. Box 649

Kealakekua, HI 96750
(808) 322-9400

Pahoa
Alan D. Thal, MD
P.O. Box 403
Pahoa, HI 96778
(808) 889-0770 FAX (808) 889-0797

IDAHO
Nampa
Stephen Thornburgh, DO
824 - 17th Ave. So.
Nampa, ID 83651
(208) 466-3517

ILLINOIS
Arlington Heights
William Mauer, DO
3401 N. Kennicott Avenue
Arlington Heights, IL 60004
(847) 255-8988 FAX (847) 255-7700

Belvidere
Oscar I. Ordonez, MD
6413 Logan Ave., #104
Belvidere, IL 61008
(815) 547-8187 FAX (815) 544-3114

Braidwood
Bernard G. Milton, MD
233 E. Reed St.
Braidwood, IL 60408
(815) 458-6700

Chicago
Alan F. Bain, DO
111 N. Wabash Ave. Ste. 1005
Chicago, IL 60602
(312) 236-7010 FAX (312) 236-7190

David Edelberg, MD
2522 N. Lincoln Avenue
Chicago, IL 60614
(773) 296-6700 FAX (773) 296-1131

Razvan Rentea, MD
3525 W. Peterson, Suite 611

Chicago, IL 60659
(773) 583-7793 FAX (773) 583-7796

Elk Grove Village
Zofia Szymanska, MD
850 Biesterfield Rd., #4006
Elk Grove Village, IL 60007
(847) 437-4418

Geneva
Richard E. Hrdlicka, MD
302 Randall Rd., #206
Geneva, IL 60134
(630) 232-1900

Hazel Crest
Prakash G. Sane, MD
17680 South Kedzie Ave.
Hazel Crest, IL 60429
(708) 799-2499 FAX (708) 799-4093

Hoffman Estates
Susan Busse, MD
Governor's Place Medical Bldg.
2260 W. Higgins Rd., #202
Hoffman Estates, IL 60195
(847) 781-7500 FAX (847) 781-7502

Metamora
Robert E. Thompson, MD
205 S. Englewood Drive
Metamora, IL 61548
(309) 367-2321 FAX (309) 367-2324

Moline
Terry W. Love, DO
2610 - 41st Street
Moline, IL 61252
(309) 764-2900

Oak Park
Paul J. Dunn, MD
715 Lake Street
Oak Park, IL 60301
(708) 383-3800 FAX (708) 383-3445

Ross A. Hauser, MD
715 Lake Street, Suite 600
Oak Park, IL 60301
(708) 848-7789 FAX (708) 848-7763

Ottawa
Terry W. Love, DO
645 W. Main Street
Ottawa, IL 61350
(815) 434-1977

Quincy
Walter Barnes, MD
3701 East Lake Centre Dr, #1
Quincy, IL 62301
(217) 224-3757 FAX (217) 224-5941

Schaumburg
Joseph Mercola, DO
1443 W. Schaumburg Rd., #250
Schaumburg, IL 60194
(847) 985-1777

Wheaton
Fred J. Schultz, MD
2150 Manchester Rd.
Wheaton, IL 60187
(630) 933-9722 FAX (630) 933-9724

INDIANA
Clarksville
Edna Pretila, MD
647 Eastern Blvd.
Clarksville, IN 47129
(812) 282-4309 FAX (812) 283-8299

George Wolverton, MD
647 Eastern Blvd.
Clarksville, IN 47129
(812) 282-4309

Evansville
Joseph Waling, MD
8601 N. Kentucky Ave., Ste. G
Evansville, IN 47725
(812) 867-9800 FAX (812) 867-4720

Goshen
Douglas W. Elliott, MD,
21764 Omega Court
Goshen, IN 46528
(574) 875-4227 FAX (574) 875-7828

Huntington
Thomas J. Ringenberg, DO
941 Etwa Avenue
Huntington, IN 46750
(219) 356-9400 FAX (219) 356-4254

Indianapolis
David R. Decatur, MD
8925 N. Meridian, #150
Indianapolis, IN 46260
(317) 818-8925

Jeffersonville
H. Wayne Mayhue, MD
207 Sparks Ave., #301
Jeffersonville, IN 47130
(812) 288-7169 FAX (812) 288-2861

Lafayette
Charles Turner, MD
2433 S. 9th Street
Lafayette, IN 47909
(765) 471-1100 FAX (765) 471-1009

Lynn
David Chopra, MD
P. O. Box 636
428 South Main St.
Lynn, IN 47355
(317) 874-2411

Merrillville
Joel F. Lopez, MD
5495 Broadway
Merrillville, IN 46410
(219) 985-5500 FAX (219) 985-5510

Mooresville
Richard N. Halstead, DO
215 E. High St.
Mooresville, IN 46158
(317) 831-0853 FAX (317) 831-0864

No. Manchester
Marvin D. Dziabis, MD
107 West Seventh Street
No. Manchester, IN 46962
(260) 982-1400 FAX (260) 982-1700

Parker City
Oscar I. Ordonez, MD
218 S. Main Street
Parker City, IN 47368
(765) 468-6337

South Bend
Larry Banyash, MD
625 East Angela Blvd.
South Bend, IN 46617
(574) 233-1533

Keim T. Houser, MD
515 N. Lafayette Blvd.
South Bend, IN 46601
(219) 232-2037

Valparaiso
Myrna D. Trowbridge, DO
850-C Marsh St.
Valparaiso, IN 46385
(219) 462-3377 FAX (219) 464-4530

Washington
Anne L. Kempf, DO
RR 3, Box 357 Bedford Road
Washington, IN 47501
(219) 232-5892

KANSAS
Coffeyville
J. E. Block, MD
1501 W. 4th
Coffeyville, KS 67337
(316) 251-2400 FAX (316) 251-1619

Garden City
Terry Hunsberger, DO
603 N. 5th. Street
Garden City, KS 67846
(316) 275-3760 FAX (316) 275-3704

Hays
Roy N. Neil, MD
105 West 13th
Hays, KS 67601
(913) 628-8341

Kansas City
Jeanne A. Drisko, MD
3901 Rainbow Blvd.
Kansas City, KS 66160
(913) 588-6208 FAX (913) 588-6271

Liberal
Bob Sager, MD
2130 N. Kansas Ave.
Liberal, KS 67901
(316) 626-5060 FAX (316) 626-7993

Topeka
John Toth, MD
2115 S.W. 10th
Topeka, KS 66604
(785) 232-3330 FAX (785) 232-1874

KENTUCKY
Berea
Edward K. Atkinson, MD
P.O. Box 57
Berea, KY 40403
(859) 925-2252 FAX (859) 925-2252

Somerset
Stephen S. Kiteck, MD
600 Bogle St.
(606) 677-0459

LOUISIANA
Alexandria
James W. Welch, MD
4300 Parliament Dr.
Alexandria, LA 71303
(318) 448-0221

Baton Rouge
Stephanie F. Cave, MD
10562 S. Glenstone Place
Baton Rouge, LA 70810
(225) 767-7433 FAX (225) 767-4641

Mark Cotter, MD
5207 Essen Lane
Baton Rouge, LA 70809
(225) 766-3171 FAX (225) 766-3271

Belle Chasse
Lawrence A. Giambelluca, MD
8200 Highway 23
Belle Chasse, LA 70037
(504) 398-1100 FAX (504) 398-1030

Chalmette
Saroj T. Tampira, MD
9000 Patricia St., Ste. 118
Chalmette, LA 70043
(504) 277-8991 FAX (504) 277-8997

Lafayette
Sydney Crackower, MD
701 Robley Dr., #100
Lafayette, LA 70503
(337) 988-4116

Norman Dykes, MD
501 W. SaintMary Blvd., #308
Lafayette, LA 70506
(337) 234-1119 FAX (337) 234-1477

Sangeeta Shah, MD
211 E. Kaliste Saloom
Lafayette, LA 70508
(337) 235-1166 FAX (337) 235-1168

Metairie
Janet Perez-Chiesa, MD
4532 W. Napoleon Ave., #210
Metairie, LA 70001
(504) 456-7539 FAX (504) 456-7542

Kashmir K. Rai, MD
4720 S. I-10 Service Rd., #305
Metairie, LA 70001
(504) 454-8952 FAX (504) 454-7708

New Orleans
James P. Carter, MD
2134 Napoleon Ave.
New Orleans, LA 70115
(504) 779-6363 FAX (504) 779-9963

MAINE
Gray
Raymond Psonak, DO
51 West Gray Rd., #1-A

P.O. Box 605
Gray, ME 04039-0605
(207) 657-4325 FAX (207) 657-4325

Portland
Alan N. Weiner, DO
4 Milk Street
Portland, ME 04101
(207) 828-8080 FAX (207) 828-6816

Waterville
Arthur Weisser, DO
81 Grove Street
Waterville, ME 04901
(207) 873-7721 FAX (207) 873-7724

MARYLAND
Annapolis
Jacob E. Teitelbaum, MD
466 Forelands Road
Annapolis, MD 21401
(410) 573-5389 FAX (410) 266-6104

Baltimore
Binyamin Rothstein, DO
2835 Smith Ave., #209
Baltimore, MD 21209
(410) 484-2121

Belcamp
Philip W. Halstead, MD
1200 Brass Mill Road
Belcamp, MD 21017
(410) 272-7751 FAX (410) 273-0476

Bethesda
Norton Fishman, MD
5413 W. Cedar Lane, #205-C
Bethesda, MD 20814
(301) 897-3599 FAX (301) 564-3116

Easton
Paul V. Beals, MD
Easton Plaza
101 Marlboro Rd., #25
Easton, MD 21601
(410) 770-5900

Laurel
Paul V. Beals, MD
9101 Cherry Lane Park, Suite 205
Laurel, MD 20708
(301) 490-9911

Lutherville
Elisabeth Lucas, MD
1205 York Road, Ste. 30A
Lutherville, MD 21093
(410) 823-3101 FAX (410) 296-0650

Kenneth B. Singleton, MD
2328 W. Joppa Rd., #310
Lutherville, MD 21093
(410) 296-3737 FAX (410) 296-0650

Stevensville
Paul V. Beals, MD
133 Log Canoe Circle
Stevensville, MD 21666
(410) 770-5900

Waldorf
F. Alexander Leon, MD
85 High Street
Waldorf, MD 20602
(301) 645-9551 FAX (301) 645-1009

MASSACHUSETTS
Arlington
Michael Janson, MD
180 Massachusetts Ave.
Arlington, MA 02474
(781) 641-1901 FAX (781) 641-3963

Glenn Rothfeld, MD
180 Massachusetts Ave., #303
Arlington, MA 02474
(781) 641-1901 FAX (781) 641-3963

Boston
Ruben Oganesov, MD
39 Brighton Ave.
Boston, MA 02134
(617) 783-5783 FAX (617) 783-1519

Earl Robert Parson, MD
495 Summer Street (MEPS)
Boston, MA 02210
(617) 753-3113

Cambridge
Leonid Gordin, MD
2500 Massachusetts Ave.
Cambridge, MA 02140
(617) 661-6225 FAX (617) 492-2002

Guy Pugh, MD
2500 Massachusetts Ave
Cambridge, MA 02140
(617) 661-6225 FAX (617) 492-2002

Vladimir P. Shurlan, MD
7 Channing St.
Cambridge, MA 02138
(617) 547-3249 FAX (617) 547-3249

Framingham
Carol Englender, MD
160 Speen Street, #203
Framingham, MA 01701
(508) 875-0875 FAX (508) 875-0005

Malden
George Milowe, MD
11 Bickford Road
Malden, MA 02148
(781) 397-7408 FAX (781) 324-2610

Newton
Jeanne Hubbuch, MD
288 Walnut Street, #420
Newton, MA 02460-1994
(617) 965-7770 FAX (617) 965-7378

Northampton
Barry D. Elson, MD
2 Maple Avenue, Ste. 52
Northampton, MA 01060
(413) 584-7787 FAX (413) 584-7778

S. Yarmouth
Paul Cochrane, DO
23-H White's Path
S. Yarmouth, MA 02664
(508) 760-2423 FAX (508) 760-1019

West Boylston
N. Thomas La Cava, MD
360 West Boylston St., Suite 107
West Boylston, MA 01583
(508) 854-1380 FAX (508) 854-1377

Winchester
Marcia Lipski, MD
9 Alben Street
Winchester, MA 01890
(508) 339-7788

MICHIGAN
Bay City
Parveen A. Malik, MD
808 N. Euclid Ave.
Bay City, MI 48706
(517) 686-3760

Clarkston
Nedra Downing, DO
5639 Sashabaw Road
Clarkston, MI 48346
(248) 625-6677 FAX (248) 625-5633

Flint
William M. Bernard, DO
1044 Gilbert Street
Flint, MI 48532
(810) 733-3140 FAX (810) 733-5623

Kenneth Ganapini, DO
1044 Gilbert Street
Flint, MI 48532
(810) 733-3140 FAX (810) 733-5623

Janice Shimoda, DO
1044 Gilbert Street
Flint, MI 48532
(810) 733-3140 FAX (810) 733-5623

Grand Rapids
Tammy Born, DO
3700 - 52nd Street S.E.
Grand Rapids, MI 49512
(616) 656-3700 FAX (616) 656-3701

Robert A. DeJonge, DO
2251 East Paris
Grand Rapids, MI 49546
(616) 956-6090 FAX (616) 956-6099

Grosse Pointe
R.B. Fahim, MD
20825 Mack Ave
Grosse Pointe, MI 48236
(313) 640-9730 FAX (313) 640-9740

Huntington Woods
Philip Hoekstra, III, PhD
26711 Woodward Ave., #203
Huntington Woods, MI 48070

Lapeer
Paul D. Lepor, DO
1254 North Main St.
Lapeer, MI 48446
(810) 664-4531

Norway
F. Michael Saigh, MD
411 Murray Rd. West U.S. 2
Norway, MI 49870
(906) 563-9600 FAX (906) 563-7110

Parchment
Eric Born, DO
2350 East G Avenue
Parchment, MI 49004
(616) 344-6183 FAX (616) 349-3046

Pontiac
Vahagn Agbabian, DO
28 No. Saginaw St., Suite 1105
Pontiac, MI 48342-2144
(248) 334-2424 FAX (248) 334-2924

Romeo
James Ziobron, DO
71441 Van Dyke
Romeo, MI 48065
(810) 336-3700 FAX (810) 336-9443

Saline
John G. Ghuneim, MD
420 Russell, #204
Saline Prof. Office Bldg.
Saline, MI 48176
(734) 429-2581 FAX (734) 429-3410

Tawas City
Michael D. Papenfuse, DO
200 Hemlock Rd.
Tawas City, MI 48764
(517) 362-9229 FAX (517) 362-9228

West Bloomfield
David Brownstein, MD
5821 W. Maple Rd., #192
West Bloomfield, MI 48322
(248) 851-1600 FAX (248) 851-0421

MINNESOTA
Minnetonka
Jean R. Eckerly, MD
13911 Ridgedale Dr., #350
Minnetonka, MN 55441
(952) 593-9458 FAX (952) 593-0097

Sortell
Tom Sult, MD
100 2nd Street S.
Sortell, MN 56377
(320) 251-2600

St. Louis Park
Michael A. Dole, MD
3408 Dakota So.
St. Louis Park, MN 55416
(612) 924-1053 FAX (612) 924-0254

St. Peter
Harold J. Fletcher, MD
220 West Broadway
St. Peter, MN 56082
(507) 934-4850 FAX (507) 934-4909

MISSISSIPPI
Coldwater
Pravin P. Patel, MD
P. O. Box 1060
Coldwater, MS 38618
(601) 622-7011

Columbus
Jacob Skiwski, MD
3491 Bluecutt Rd.
Columbus, MS 39701
(601) 329-2955 or 327-0646

Ocean Springs
James H. Waddell, MD
1520 Government Street
Ocean Springs, MS 39564
(228) 875-5505

MISSOURI

Kansas City
Edward McDonagh, DO
2800-A Kendallwood Pkwy.
Kansas City, MO 64119
(816) 453-5940 FAX (816) 453-1140

Charles Rudolph, DO
2800-A Kendallwood Pkwy.
Kansas City, MO 64119
(816) 453-5940 FAX (816) 453-1140

Springfield
Neil Nathan, MD
2828 N. National, #D
Springfield, MO 65803
(417) 869-7583 FAX (417) 869-7592

William Sunderwirth, DO
2828 N. National
Springfield, MO 65803
(417) 837-4158

St. Louis
Lena R. Capapas, MD
3009 N. Ballas Rd., #132-A
St. Louis, MO 63131
(314) 995-9713 FAX (314) 995-9818

Octavio R. Chirino, MD
9701 Landmark Pkwy. Dr., #207
St. Louis, MO 63127
(314) 842-4802

Varsha Rathod, MD
1977 Schuetz Rd.
St. Louis, MO 63146
(314) 997-5403 FAX (314) 997-6837

Simon M. Yu, MD
11710 Old Ballas Rd., #205
St. Louis, MO 63141
(314) 432-7802 FAX (314) 432-1971

MONTANA

Billings
David C. Healow, MD
2501 - 4th Avenue North, #C
Billings, MT 59101-1317
(406) 252-6674

Bozeman
Curt Kurtz, MD
300 N. Willson, #502E
Bozeman, MT 59715
(406) 587-5561 FAX (406) 585-8536

Great Falls
Bonnie Friehling, MD
2517 7th Avenue South, #B-3
Great Falls, MT 59405
(406) 761-5778 FAX (406) 761-7117

NEBRASKA

Hartington
Steve Vlach, MD
405 W. Darlene St., P.O. Box 937
Hartington, NE 68739
(402) 254-3935 FAX (402) 254-2393

North Platte
Loretta Baca, MD
302 S. Jeffers St.
North Platte, NE 69103
(308) 534-6687 FAX (308) 534-1874

Omaha
James Murphy, Jr., DO
8031 W. Center Road, #221
Omaha, NE 68124
(402) 343-7963 FAX (402) 343-1330

Eugene C. Oliveto, MD
10804 Prairie Hills Dr.
Omaha, NE 68144
(402) 392-0233

Jeffrey Passer, MD
9300 Underwood Ave., Suite 520
Omaha, NE 68114
(402) 398-1200 FAX (402) 398-9119

NEVADA

Carson City
Frank Shallenberger, MD
896 W. Nye Lane, #103
Carson City, NV 89703
(775) 884-3990 FAX (775) 884-2202

Henderson
Hector R. Fernandez, MD
1673 Black Fox Canyon Rd.
Henderson, NV 89052

Dan F. Royal, DO
2501 N. Green Valley Pkwy.,
#D-132
Henderson, NV 89014
(702) 433-8800 FAX (702) 433-8823

Las Vegas
Steven Holper, MD
3233 W. Charleston, #202
Las Vegas, NV 89102
(702) 878-3510 FAX (702) 878-1405

Robert D. Milne, MD
2110 Pinto Lane
Las Vegas, NV 89106
(702) 385-1393 FAX (702) 385-4170

Adelaida Resuello, MD
1300 S. Maryland Pkwy.
Las Vegas, NV 89104
(702) 367-2107 FAX (702) 367-6554

F. Fuller Royal, MD
3663 Pecos McLeod
Las Vegas, NV 89121
(702) 732-1400 FAX (702) 732-9661

Reno
W. Douglas Brodie, MD
601 West Moana Lane
Reno, NV 89509
(775) 829-1009 FAX (775) 829-9330

Hector de los Santos, MD
6490 S. McCarran Blvd., #D-41
Reno, NV 89509
(775) 827-6696

David A. Edwards, MD
6490 S. McCarran Bl., #C-24
Reno, NV 89509
(775) 827-1444 FAX (775) 827-2424

Michael L. Gerber, MD
3670 Grant Dr., #101
Reno, NV 89509
(775) 826-1900

Corazon Ibarra, MD
6490 S. McCarran Blvd., #D-41
Reno, NV 89509
(775) 827-1444 FAX (775) 827-2424

Corazon Ibarra-Ilarina, MD
6490 S. McCarran Blvd., #C-24
Reno, NV 89509
(775) 827-1444 FAX (775) 827-2424

NEW JERSEY
Bloomfield
Majid Ali, MD
320 Belleville Ave.
Bloomfield, NJ 07003
(973) 586-4111

Richard L. Podkul, MD
1064 Broad Street
Bloomfield, NJ 07003
(973) 893-0282 FAX (973) 893-0612

Brick
Ivan Krohn, MD
1140 Burnt Tavern Road
Brick, NJ 08724
(732) 785-2670 FAX (732) 785-2673

Brigantine
Michael J. Dunn, MD
1311 East Shove Drive
Brigantine, NJ 08203
(609) 266-0400 FAX (609) 266-2597

Cedar Grove
Robert Steinfeld, MD
912 Pompton Ave., #9-B-1
Canfield Ofc.Pk.
Cedar Grove, NJ 07009
(973) 243-9898 FAX (973) 835-8312

Cherry Hill
Scott R. Greenberg, MD
1907 Greentree Rd.
Cherry Hill, NJ 08003
(856) 424-8222 FAX (856) 424-2599

Allan Magaziner, DO
1907 Greentree Road
Cherry Hill, NJ 08003
(856) 424-8222 FAX (856) 424-2599

Denville
Majid Ali, MD
95 E. Main Street, #101
Denville, NJ 07834
(973) 586-4111 FAX (973) 586-8466

Edison
Richard B. Menashe, DO
15 South Main St.
Edison, NJ 08837
(732) 906-8866 FAX (732) 906-0124

James Neubrander, MD
15 S. Main Street, #6
Edison, NJ 08837
(732) 634-3666 FAX (732) 634-8008

Herbert Smyczek, MD
668 Grove Avenue
Edison, NJ 08820-3225
(732) 548-5432

Elizabeth
Gennaro Locurcio, MD
610 Third Avenue
Elizabeth, NJ 07202
(908) 351-1333 FAX (908) 351-3740

Fair Lawn
Anthony M. Giliberti, DO
14-01 Broadway
Fair Lawn, NJ 07410
(201) 797-8534

Forked River
Mark J. Bartiss, MD
933 Lacey Road
Forked River, NJ 08050
(609) 693-2000

Fort Lee
Gary Klingsberg, DO
1355 15th Street, #200
Fort Lee, NJ 07024
(201) 585-9368 FAX (201) 585-0162

Hackensack
Robin Leder, MD
235 Prospect Ave.
Hackensack, NJ 07601
(201) 525-1155

Haddonfield
Roberta Morgan, DO
30 N. Haddon Ave.
Haddonfield, NJ 08033-2429
(856) 216-9001 FAX (856) 616-9837

Lakewood
Gloria Freundlich, DO
122 Hope Chapel Road
Lakewood, NJ 08701
(732) 961-9217

Manasquan
Vladimir Berkovich, MD
1707 Atlantic Ave., Bldg. B
Manasquan, NJ 08736
(732) 292-2101 FAX (732) 292-2105

Middletown
David Dornfeld, DO
18 Leonardville Rd.
Middletown, NJ 07748
(732) 671-3730 FAX (732) 706-1078

Neil Rosen, DO
18 Leonardville Rd.
Middletown, NJ 07748
(732) 671-3730 FAX (732) 706-1078

Millburn
Sharda Sharma, MD
131 Millburn Avenue
Millburn, NJ 07041
(973) 376-4500 FAX (973) 467-2285

Daniel Zacharias, MD
68 Essex Street
Millburn, NJ 07041
(973) 912-0006 FAX (973) 912-0007

Millville
Charles Mintz, MD
10 E. Broad Street
Millville, NJ 08332
(609) 825-7372 FAX (609) 327-6588

Morris Plains
David M. Strassberg, MD
27 Fernview Road
Morris Plains, NJ 07950
(732) 855-7700

Morristown
Faina Munits, MD
4 Boxwood Drive
Morristown, NJ 07960-4545
(973) 292-3222 FAX (973) 292-3443

Newark
Stephen Holt, MD
105 Lock Street, Ste. 405
Newark, NJ 07103
(973) 824-8800 FAX (973) 824-8822

North Wildwood
John G. Costino, DO
404 Surf Avenue
North Wildwood, NJ 08260
(609) 522-8358 FAX (609) 729-8662

Northfield
Barry D. Glasser, MD
1907 New Road
Northfield, NJ 08225
(609) 646-9600 FAX (609) 484-8127

Paramus
Thomas A. Cacciola, MD
403 Farview Ave.
Paramus, NJ 07652
(201) 261-8386 FAX (201) 261-8827

Redbank
Dominick Grosso, DO
5 Globe Ct.
Redbank, NJ 07701
(732) 219-0110 FAX (732) 212-8818

Ridgewood
Arie Rave, MD
1250 E. Ridgewood Ave.
Ridgewood, NJ 07450
(201) 689-1900 FAX (201) 447-9011

Stuart Weg, MD
1250 E. Ridgewood Ave.
Ridgewood, NJ 07450
(201) 447-5558 FAX (201) 447-9011

Roselle Park
Yulius Poplyansky, MD
236 E. Westfield Avenue

Roselle Park, NJ 07204
(908) 241-3800 FAX (908) 241-9668

Shrewsbury
David Dornfeld, DO
555 Shrewsbury Ave.
Shrewsbury, NJ 07702
(732) 219-0894 FAX (732) 219-0896

Neil Rosen, DO
555 Shrewsbury Ave.
Shrewsbury, NJ 07702
(732) 219-0894 FAX (732) 219-0896

Somerset
Marc Condren, MD
7 Cedar Grove Lane, #20
Somerset, NJ 08873
(908) 469-2133

Stockton
Stuart H. Freedenfeld, MD
56 So. Main St., #A
Stockton, NJ 08559
(609) 397-8585 FAX (609) 397-9335

Trenton
Imtiaz Ahmad, MD
1760 Whitehorse Hamilton Sq. Rd.,
#5
Trenton, NJ 08690
(609) 890-2966 FAX (609) 890-3326

Robert J. Peterson, DO
2239 Whitehorse/Mercerville Rd.,
#4
Trenton, NJ 08619
(215) 579-0330

Union City
Michael J. Calache, MD
4418 Kennedy Blvd.
Union City, NJ 07087
(201) 863-3111

Simon Santos, MD
410 - 36th Street
Union City, NJ 07087
(201) 863-7744 FAX (201) 863-7608

NEW MEXICO
Albuquerque
Ralph J. Luciani, DO
10601 Lomas Blvd. NE, #103
Albuquerque, NM 87112
(505) 298-5995 FAX (505) 298-2940

Las Cruces
Burton M. Berkson, MD, PhD
741 N. Alameda, #12
Las Cruces, NM 88005
(505) 524-3720 FAX (505) 521-1815

Wolfgang Haese, MD
4105 N. Main Street
Las Cruces, NM 88012
(505) 373-8415 FAX (505) 373-8416

Santa Fe
Shirley B. Scott, MD
P. O. Box 2670
Santa Fe, NM 87504
(505) 986-9960

W. A. Shrader, Jr., MD
141 Paseo de Peralta
Santa Fe, NM 87501
(505) 983-8890 FAX (505) 820-7315

NEW YORK
Albany
Kenneth A. Bock, MD
10 McKown RD
Pinnacle Place, Suite 210
Albany, NY 12203
(518) 435-0082 FAX (518) 435-0086

Albertson
Steven Rachlin, MD
927 Willis Avenue
Albertson, L.I., NY 11507
(516) 873-7773 FAX (516) 877-7365

Brewster
Jeffrey C. Kopelson, MD
221 Clock Tower Commons
Brewster, NY 10509
(914) 278-6800 FAX (914) 278-6897

Bronx
Richard Izquierdo, MD
1070 Southern Blvd., Lower Level
Bronx, NY 10459
(718) 589-4541

Bronxville
Joseph S. Wojcik, MD
525 Bronxville Rd.,1-G
Bronxville, NY 10708
(914) 793-6161

Brooklyn
Gloria W. Freundlich, DO
575 Ocean Parkway
Brooklyn, NY 11218
(718) 437-4459

Levi H. Lehv, MD
6910 Avenue U
Brooklyn, NY 11234
(718) 251-1200

Igor Ostrovsky, MD
3120 Brighton 5th Street, # 1-C
Brooklyn, NY 11235
(718) 934-1920 FAX (718) 934-2078

Michael Teplitsky, MD
415 Oceanview Ave.
Brooklyn, NY 11235
(718) 769-0997 FAX (718) 646-2352

Pavel Yutsis, MD
264 1st Street
Brooklyn, NY 11215
(718) 621-0900 FAX (718) 621-9165

Buffalo
Kalpana Patel, MD
65 Wehrle Drive
Buffalo, NY 14225
(716) 833-2213 FAX (716) 833-2244

Chappaqua
Savely Yurkovsky, MD
37 King Street
Chappaqua, NY 10514
(914) 861-9161

East Meadow
Kathryn Calabria, DO
30 Merrick Ave., #111
East Meadow, NY 11554
(516) 542-9090 FAX (516) 542-9258

Fredonia
Robert F. Barnes, DO
3489 E. Main Rd.
Fredonia, NY 14063
(716) 679-3510 FAX (716) 679-3512

Glens Falls
Ann Auburn, DO
15 W. Notre Dame Street
Glens Falls, NY 12801
(518) 745-7473 FAX (518) 792-7310

Andrew W. Garner, MD
8 Harrison Avenue
Glens Falls, NY 12801
(518) 798-9401 FAX (518) 798-9411

Hamburg
Robert F. Barnes, DO
5225 Southwestern Blvd.
Hamburg, NY 14075
(716) 649-0225 FAX (716) 649-0369

Ronald P. Santasiero, MD
5451 Southwestern Blvd.
Hamburg, NY 14075
(716) 646-6075 FAX (716) 646-5912

Islip
John P. Salerno, DO
72 Marina Way
Islip, NY 11751
(352) 237-1103 FAX (352) 861-5447

Lake Success
Maurice Cohen, MD
2 ProHealth Plaza
Lake Success, NY 11042
(516) 608-2806 FAX (516) 608-2805

Lawrence
Mitchell Kurk, MD
310 Broadway
Lawrence, NY 11559
(516) 239-5540 FAX (516) 371-2919

Lewiston
Donald M. Fraser, MD
5147 Lewiston Rd.
Lewiston, NY 14092
(716) 284-5777

Merrick
Susan Groh, MD
2916 Frankel Blvd.
Merrick, NY 11566
(516) 867-5132 FAX (516) 867-5519

Middletown
Levi H. Lehv, MD
825 Route 211 East
Middletown, NY 10941
(914) 692-8338 FAX (914) 692-6177

Mt. Kisco
Michael Finkelstein, MD
400 East Main Street
Mt. Kisco, NY 10549
(914) 666-1308 FAX (914) 666-1965

Neil C. Raff, MD
213 Main Street
Mt. Kisco, NY 10549
(914) 241-7030

New City
Arthur Landau, MD
10 Esquire Road
New City, NY 10956
(914) 638-4464 FAX (914) 638-4509

New Rochelle
Harold C. Clark, MD
400 Webster Ave.
New Rochelle, NY 10801
(914) 235-8385

New York
Richard N. Ash, MD
800-A Fifth Ave. 61st St.
New York, NY 10021
(212) 758-3200 FAX (212) 754-5800

Robert C. Atkins, MD
152 E. 55th St.
New York, NY 10022
(212) 758-2110 FAX (212) 751-1863

Thomas Bolte, MD
141 East 55th Street, #8H
New York, NY 10022
(212) 588-9314 FAX (212) 702-9856

Eric R. Braverman, MD
185 Madison Ave., 6th floor
New York, NY 10016-4325
(212) 213-6155 FAX (212) 213-6188

Claudia M. Cooke, MD
133 East 73rd Street, #506
New York, NY 10021
(212) 861-9000 FAX (212) 585-4177

Ronald Hoffman, MD
40 E. 30th Street
New York, NY 10016
(212) 779-1744 FAX (212) 779-0891

Warren Levin, MD
31 East 28th Street, 6th Flr.
New York, NY 10016
(212) 679-9667 FAX (212) 679-9730

Gennaro Locurcio, MD
112 Lexington Avenue
New York, NY 10016
(212) 696-2680 FAX (212) 696-2694

Jeffrey A. Morrison, MD
40 E. 30th Street, 10th Floor
New York, NY 10016
(212) 779-1744 FAX (212) 779-0891

Fred Pescatore, MD
274 Madison Avenue, #402
New York, NY 10016
(212) 779-2944 FAX (212) 223-9757

Francesca Skolas, MD
200 Park Ave. South, 3rd Floor
New York, NY 10003
(212) 780-4459 FAX (212) 420-7211

Michael J. Teplitsky, MD
31 East 28 Street
New York, NY 10016
(212) 679-3700 FAX (212) 679-9730

Lawrence Young, MD
19 Bowery Street, Rm. 1
New York, NY 10002-6702
(212) 431-4343 FAX (212) 925-8637

Niagara Falls
Paul Cutler, MD
652 Elmwood Ave.
Niagara Falls, NY 14301
(716) 284-5140 FAX (716) 284-5159

Orangeburg
Neil L. Block, MD
14 Prel Plaza
Orangeburg, NY 10962
(914) 359-3300

Rhinebeck
Kenneth A. Bock, MD
108 Montgomery St.
Rhinebeck, NY 12572
(845) 876-7082 FAX (845) 876-4615

Steven Bock, MD
108 Montgomery Street
Rhinebeck, NY 12572
(845) 876-7082 FAX (845) 876-4615

Rochester
Paul Cutler, MD
1081 Long Pond Rd.
Rochester, NY 14626
(585) 720-1980

Suffern
Michael B. Schachter, MD
Two Executive Blvd., #202
Suffern, NY 10901
(845) 368-4700 FAX (845) 368-4727

Utica
Richard O'Brien, DO
2305 Genesee Street
Utica, NY 13501
(315) 724-8888

Margarita Schilling, MD
2305 Genesee Street
Utica, NY 13501
(315) 797-3799 FAX (315) 734-1912

Woodside
Fira Nihamin, MD
39 - 65 52nd Street
Woodside, NY 11377
(718) 429-0039 FAX (718) 429-6965

NORTH CAROLINA

Asheville
James Biddle, MD
239 S. French Broad Ave.
Asheville, NC 28801
(828) 252-5545 FAX (828) 281-3055

Ronald Parks, MD
801 Fairview Road, #142
Asheville, NC 28803
(828) 298-7638 FAX (828) 296-0578

John L. Wilson Jr., MD
Park Terrace Center, 1312
Patton Ave.
Asheville, NC 28806
(828) 252-9833 FAX (828) 255-8118

Eileen M. Wright, MD
Park Terrace Center, 1312
Patton Ave.
Asheville, NC 28806
(828) 252-9833 FAX (828) 255-8118

Carolina Beach
Keith E. Johnson, MD
1009 N. Lake Park Blvd., Box 16,
C-5
Pleasure Island Plaza
Carolina Beach, NC 28428
(910) 458-0606

Charlotte
Rashid Ali Buttar, DO
20721 Torrence Chapel, #101
Charlotte, NC 28031
(704) 895-9355 FAX (704) 895-9357

Tyler Freeman, MD
3135 Springbank Lane, #100
Charlotte, NC 28226
(704) 716-7979 FAX (704) 523-5453

Mark O'Neal Speight, MD
2317 Randolph Rd.
Charlotte, NC 28207
(704) 334-8447 FAX (704) 334-0733

Fletcher (Asheville)
Stephen Blievernicht, MD
242 Old Concord Rd.

Fletcher (Asheville), NC 28732
(828) 684-4411 FAX (828) 684-7657

Hillsborough
Dennis W. Fera, MD
1000 Corporate Dr., #209
Hillsborough (Chapel Hill), NC
27278
(919) 732-2287 FAX (919) 732-3176

Mooresville
Anthony J. Castiglia, MD
570 Williamson Road, Ste. C
Mooresville, NC 28117
(704) 799-9740 FAX (704) 799-9742

Morehead City
Donald Brooks Reece II, MD
#2 Medical Park
Morehead City, NC 28557
(252) 247-5177 FAX (252) 247-0223

Murphy
Robert E. Moreland, MD
75 Medical Park Lane, #C
Murphy, NC 28906
(828) 837-7997

Raleigh
John C. Pittman, MD
4505 Fair Meadow Lane, #111
Raleigh, NC 27607
(919) 571-4391 FAX (919) 571-8968

Thomas Spruill, MD
3900 Browning Place, #201
Raleigh, NC 27609
(919) 787-7125 FAX (919) 787-9952

Roanoke Rapids
Bhaskar D. Power, MD
1201 E. Littleton Rd.
Roanoke Rapids, NC 27870
(252) 535-1412

Rocky Mount
Lemuel Kornegay, MD
500 Shady Circle
Rocky Mount, NC 27803
(252) 442-7017 FAX (252) 442-5022

Southern Pines
Keith E. Johnson, MD
1852 U.S. Hwy. 1 South
Southern Pines, NC 28387
(910) 695-0335 FAX (910) 695-3697

Tryon
Mack Stuart Bonner Jr, MD
590 South Trade Street
Tryon, NC 28782
(828) 859-0420 FAX (828) 859-0422

Connie G. Ross, MD
590 South Trade Street
Tryon, NC 28782
(828) 859-0420 FAX (828) 859-0422

Winston-Salem
Walter Ward, MD
1411B Plaza West Road
(336) 760-0240 FAX (336) 760-4568

Laurence Webster, MD
2803 Lyndhurst Ave.
Winston-Salem, NC 27103
(336) 499-3800

NORTH DAKOTA
Grand Forks
Richard H. Leigh, MD
2600 Demers Ave., #108
Grand Forks, ND 58201
(701) 772-7696

Minot
Brian E. Briggs, MD
718 - 6th Street S.W.
Minot, ND 58701
(701) 838-6011 FAX (701) 838-5055

OHIO
Akron
Josephine C. Aronica, MD
1867 W. Market St.
Akron, OH 44313
(330) 867-7361 FAX (330) 867-7362

Bluffton
L. Terry Chappell, MD
122 Thurman St. - Box 248

Bluffton, OH 45817
(419) 358-4627 FAX (419) 358-1855

Centerville
John Boyles, Jr., MD
7076 Corporate Way
Centerville, OH 45459
(513) 434-0555

Cincinnati
Kaushal K. Bhardwaj, MD
9019 Colerain Ave.
Cincinnati, OH 45251
(513) 385-8100 FAX (513) 385-8106

Ted Cole, DO
11974 Lebanon Rd., Ste. 228
Cincinnati, OH 45241
(513) 779-0300

Leonid Macheret, MD
375 Glensprings Dr., #400
Cincinnati, OH 45246
(513) 851-8790 FAX (513) 851-0434

James E. Smith, DO
11263 Reading Road
Cincinnati, OH 45241
(513) 769-7546 FAX (513) 769-7547

Cleveland
Radha Baishnab, MD
5599 Pearl Rd.
Cleveland, OH 44129-2544
(440) 234-8080 FAX (440) 234-0525

John M. Baron, DO
4807 Rockside, Ste. 100
Cleveland, OH 44131
(216) 642-0082 FAX (216) 642-1415

James P. Frackelton, MD
24700 Center Ridge Rd.
Cleveland, OH 44145
(440) 835-0104 FAX (440) 871-1404

Stan Gardner, MD
24700 Center Ridge Rd.
Cleveland, OH 44145
(440) 835-0104 FAX (440) 871-1404

Derrick Lonsdale, MD
24700 Center Ridge Rd.

Cleveland, OH 44145
(440) 835-0104 FAX (440) 871-1404

Columbus
Larry S. Everhart, MD
730 Mt. Airyshire
Columbus, OH 43235
(614) 848-2600 FAX (614) 888-3938

Bruce A. Massau, DO
1492 E. Broad St., #1203
Columbus, OH 43205-1546
(614) 252-1500 FAX (614) 252-1685

Lancaster
Jacqueline S. Chan, DO
3484 Cincinnati Zanesville Rd.
Lancaster, OH 43130
(740) 653-0017 FAX (740) 653-8707

Mansfield
Ho Young Chung, MD
517 Park Ave. East, #B
Mansfield, OH 44905-2871
(419) 589-8819 FAX (419) 589-8820

Paulding
Don K. Snyder, MD
1030 West Wayne Street
Paulding, OH 45879
(419) 399-2045

Powell
Richard Ray Mason, DO
10034 Brewster Lane
Powell, OH 43065
(614) 761-0555 FAX (614) 761-8937

William D. Mitchell, DO
10034 Brewster Ln.
Powell, OH 43065-7571
(614) 761-0555 FAX (614) 761-8937

Sandusky
Douglas Weeks, MD
3703 Columbus Avenue
Sandusky, OH 44870
(419) 625-8085

Toledo
James C. Roberts Jr., MD
4607 Sylvania Ave., #200
Toledo, OH 43623
(419) 882-9620 FAX (419) 882-9628

Xenia
James E. Smith, DO
2380 Bellbrook Avenue
Xenia, OH 45385

Youngstown
James Ventresco Jr., DO
3848 Tippecanoe Rd.
Youngstown, OH 44511
(330) 792-2349

OKLAHOMA
Broken Arrow
R. Jeff Wright, DO
5050 E. Kenosha
Broken Arrow, OK 74014
(918) 496-5444 FAX (918) 496-5445

Jenks
Gerald Wootan, DO
715 West Main St., #S
Jenks, OK 74037
(918) 299-9447

Oklahoma City
Adam Merchant, MD
3535 N.W. 58th Street
Oklahoma City, OK 73112
(405) 942-8346 FAX (405) 942-8347

Charles D. Taylor, MD
4409 Classen Blvd.
Oklahoma City, OK 73118
(405) 525-7751 FAX (405) 525-0303

Ray E. Zimmer, DO
5419 S. Western Ave.
Oklahoma City, OK 73109
(405) 634-7855 FAX (405) 634-0778

Pawnee
Gordon P. Laird, DO
304 Boulder

Pawnee, OK 74058
(918) 762-3601 FAX (918) 762-2544

Valliant
Ray E. Zimmer, DO
602 No. Dalton
Valliant, OK 74764
(580) 933-4235

OREGON
Ashland
Franklin H. Ross Jr, MD
565 A Street
Ashland, OR 97520
(541) 482-7007 FAX (541) 482-5123

Bend
Chris Hatlestad, MD
2195 NE Professional Ct.
Bend, OR 97701
(541) 388-3804

Eugene
John Gambee, MD
66 Club Road, #140
Eugene, OR 97401
(541) 686-2536 FAX (541) 686-2349

Klamath Falls
Robert P. Beaman, MD
1903 Austin St., #B
Klamath Falls, OR 97603
(541) 885-9989 FAX (541) 885-7998

Medford
Helen Trew, MD
2921 Doctor's Park Drive
Medford, OR 97504
(541) 770-1143 FAX (541) 772-9149

Portland
Richard C. Heitsch, MD
171 N.E. 102nd Avenue
Professional Plaza 102, Bldg. V
Portland, OR 97220
(503) 257-3327 FAX (503) 257-3374

Jay A. Mead, MD
4444 SW Corbett Avenue

Portland, OR 97201
(503) 224-4003 FAX (503) 224-4854

David J. Ogle, MD
177 NE 102nd Avenue, Bldg. V
Portland, OR 97220
(503) 261-0966 FAX (503) 252-2697

Jeffrey Tyler, MD
163 N.E. 102nd Ave.
Portland, OR 97220
(503) 255-4256

Salem
Terence Howe Young, MD
1205 Wallace Rd. NW
Salem, OR 97304
(503) 371-1558

Springfield
S. Kathleen Hirtz, MD
1800 Centennial Blvd., #6
Springfield, OR 97477
(541) 726-1865 FAX (541) 726-2179

PENNSYLVANIA
Bangor
Francis J. Cinelli, DO
153 N. 11th Street
Bangor, PA 18013
(610) 588-4502 FAX (610) 588-6928

Bensalem
Robert J. Peterson, DO
2169 Galloway Rd.
Bensalem, PA 19020
(215) 579-0330

Bethlehem
Sally Ann Rex, DO
1343 Easton Ave.
Bethlehem, PA 18018
(610) 866-0900 FAX (610) 866-8333

Darby
Lance Wright, MD
112 S. 4th Street
Darby, PA 19023
(610) 461-6225 FAX (610) 583-3356

Doylestown
Steven C. Halbert, MD
Medical Healing Arts Center
52 East Oakland Ave.
Doylestown, PA 18901
(215) 348-4002 FAX (215) 887-1921

Erie
Karl J. Falk, DO
4234 Buffalo Rd.
Erie, PA 16510
(814) 899-7777 FAX (814) 899-1945

Exton
Ronald P. Ciccone, MD
Baxter Business Ctr. II
4995 Thomas Jones Way, Suite 202
Exton, PA 19341
(610) 594-5502 FAX (610) 594-1017

Farrell
Robert D. Multari, DO
2120 Likens Lane, #101
Farrell, PA 16121
(412) 981-3731 FAX (412) 981-3740

Fountainville
Harold H. Byer, MD, PhD
5045 Swamp Rd., #A-101
Fountainville, PA 18923
(215) 348-0443 FAX (215) 348-9124

Greensburg
Ralph A. Miranda, MD
RD. #12 - Box 108
Greensburg, PA 15601
(724) 838-7632 FAX (724) 836-3655

Hazelton
Martin Mulders, MD
53 West Juniper Street
Hazelton, PA 18201
(570) 455-4704 FAX (570) 455-4706

Hershey
Adrian J. Hohenwarter, MD
326 W. Chocolate Ave.
Hershey, PA 17033
(717) 534-2481 FAX (717) 533-2442

Jeannette
R. Christopher Monsour, MD
70 Lincoln Way East
Monsour Medical Center
Jeannette, PA 15644
(412) 527-1511

Jeffersonville
Anthony J. Bazzan, MD
2505 Blvd. Of Generals
Jeffersonville, PA 19403
(610) 630-8600 FAX (610) 630-9599

Lower Burrell
Louis K. Hauber, MD
2533 Leechburg Rd.
Lower Burrell, PA 15680
(724) 334-0966 FAX (724) 339-4223

Manheim
Kenneth F. Lovell, DO
76 Doe Run Road
Manheim, PA 17545
(717) 665-6400 (717) 664-4793

Mechanicsburg
John M. Sullivan, MD
1001 S. Market St., #B
Mechanicsburg, PA 17055
(717) 697-5050 FAX (717) 697-3156

Media
Arthur K. Balin, MD
110 Chesley Drive
Media, PA 19063
(610) 565-3300 FAX (610) 565-9909

Mt. Pleasant
Mamduh El-Attrache, MD
20 E. Main St.
Mt. Pleasant, PA 15666
(412) 547-3576

Narberth
Andrew Lipton, DO
822 Montgomery Ave., #315
Narberth, PA 19072
(610) 667-4601 FAX (610) 667-6416

Newtown
Robert J. Peterson, DO
1614 Wrightstown Rd.
Newtown, PA 18940
(215) 579-0330

North Wales
Domenick Braccia, DO
1146 Stump Road
North Wales, PA 19454
(215) 368-2160

Paoli
Martin Mulders, MD
18 Paoli Pike, 1st Floor
Paoli, PA 19301
(610) 725-9996 FAX (610) 725-9997

Penndel
Eric R. Braverman, MD
142 Bellevue Ave.
Penndel, PA 19047
(215) 702-1344 FAX (215) 757-1707

George Danielewski, MD
142 Bellevue Ave.
Penndel, PA 19047
(215) 757-4455

Philadelphia
John Bowden, DO
1738 W. Cheltenham
P.O. Box 14299
Philadelphia, PA 19138
(215) 548-3390 FAX (215) 549-8998

George Danielewski, MD
7927 Fairfield St.
Philadelphia, PA 19152
(215) 338-8866

Sarah M. Fisher, MD
530 South 2nd St., #108
Philadelphia, PA 19147
(215) 627-3001 FAX (215) 627-0362

Alan F. Kwon, MD
211 South Street, #345
Philadelphia, PA 19147
(215) 629-5633 FAX (215) 629-5633

Patrick J. Lariccia, MD
51 N. 39th Street
Philadelphia, PA 19104-2640
(215) 662-8988 FAX (215) 662-8859

Robert Smith, MD
1420 Locust Street, #200
Philadelphia, PA 19102
(215) 545-2828

Pittsburgh
Dominic A. Brandy, MD
2275 Swallow Hill Road, #2400
Pittsburgh, PA 15220
(412) 429-1151 FAX (412) 429-0211

Arthur David, MD
120 Marion Street
Pittsburgh, PA 15219
(412) 232-3555 FAX (412) 734-5885

David Goldstein, MD
9401 McKnight Rd., #301-B
Pittsburgh, PA 15237
(412) 366-6780

Edward C. Kondrot, MD
20 Cedar Blvd., Ste. 303
Pittsburgh, PA 15228
(602) 652-9285

Quakertown
Harold Buttram, MD
5724 - Clymer Road
Quakertown, PA 18951
(215) 536-1890

William G. Kracht, DO
5724 Clymer Rd.
Quakertown, PA 18951
(215) 536-1890

Scranton
Kyung Lee, MD
1027 Pittston Ave.
Scranton, PA 18505
(570) 961-0200

Okhee Won, MD
1822 Mulberry St.
Scranton, PA 18510
(570) 969-8165 FAX (570) 969-8729

Springfield
Walter W. Schwartz, DO
471 Baltimore Pike
Springfield, PA 19064
(610) 604-4800 FAX (610) 604-4815

Topton
Conrad Maulfair, Jr., DO
403 N. Main St., P.O.Box 98
Topton, PA 19562
(610) 682-2104 FAX (610) 682-9781

West Middlesex
Robert D. Multari, DO
15 Elliott Rd.
West Middlesex, PA 16159
(412) 981-2246

Williamsport
Francis M. Powers, Jr., MD
1201 Grampian Blvd., #3-A
3rd floor
Williamsport, PA 17701
(570) 322-6450 FAX (570) 322-0648

RHODE ISLAND
Greenville
Zofia Laszewski, MD
3 W. Prospect Street
Greenville, RI 02828
(401) 949-2334

Newport
Dariusz J. Nasiek, MD
17 Friendship Street
Newport, RI 02840
(401) 846-1230

SOUTH CAROLINA
Beaufort
Kenneth Orbeck, DO
9A Rue Du Bois Rd.
Beaufort, SC 29902
(843) 322-8050 FAX (842) 322-8059

Charleston
Art M. LaBruce, MD
9231A Medical Plaza Dr.

N. Charleston, SC 29406
(843) 572-1771 FAX (843) 572-8962

Columbia
James M. Shortt, MD
3981 Edmund Hwy., #A
W. Columbia, SC 29170
(803) 755-0114 FAX (803) 755-0116

Greenville
Steven R. Buckholz, DO
609 Cleveland Street
Greenville, SC 29601
(864) 233-2764 FAX (864) 271-7342

Myrtle Beach
Donald Tice, DO
4301 Highway 544
Myrtle Beach, SC 29588
(803) 215-5000 FAX (803) 215-5005

SOUTH DAKOTA
Custer
Dennis R. Wicks, MD
1 Holiday Trail, HCR 83, Box 21
Custer, SD 57730-9703
(605) 673-2689

Sioux Falls
Harold J. Fletcher, MD
4601 S. Techlink Circle
Sioux Falls, SD 57106
(605) 362-8256 FAX (605) 362-8293

TENNESSEE
Athens
H. Joseph Holliday, MD
1005 W. Madison Ave.
Athens, TN 37303
(423) 744-7540 FAX (423) 745-4898

Chattanooga
Charles C. Adams, MD
600 W. Main Street
Chattanooga, TN 37402
(706) 861-7377 FAX (706) 861-7922

Cleveland
Charles C. Adams, MD
2600 Executive Park Dr. NW
Cleveland, TN 37311
(423) 473-7080 FAX (413)473 7780

Charles C. Adams, MD
Bradley Executive Plaza
1510 Stuart Road, Ste. 106
Cleveland, TN 37312
(423) 472-1456 FAX (423) 472-1150

Hixson
Mark T. Simpson, MD
4513 Hixon Pike, #102
Hixson, TN 37343
(423) 877-7999 FAX (423) 877-7901

Kingsport
Pickens Gantt, MD
#307 - 2204 Pavilion Dr.
Kingsport, TN 37660
(423) 392-6330 FAX (423) 392-6053

David Livingston, MD
1567 N. Eastman Rd., #4
Kingsport, TN 37604
(423) 245-6671 FAX (423) 245-0966

Knoxville
Joseph Rich, MD
9217 Parkwest Blvd., #E-1
Knoxville, TN 37923
(865) 934-0133 FAX (865) 694-7658

Memphis
Jerry R. Floyd, MD
1027 Whitney Ave.
Memphis, TN 38127
(901) 353-5009 FAX (901) 353-6549

Charles Wallace, Jr., MD
1325 Eastmoreland Ave., #425
Memphis, TN 38104
(901) 272-3200 FAX (901) 278-3441

Morristown
Donald Thompson, MD
1121 W. First North St.
Morristown, TN 37816-2088
(423) 581-6367

Nashville
Stephen L. Reisman, MD
2325 Crestmoor Rd., #P-150
Nashville, TN 37215
(615) 298-2820 FAX (615) 298-2770

Old Hickory
Russell Hunt, MD
1415 Robinson Road
Old Hickory, TN 37138
(615) 541-0400 FAX (615) 847-4142

White Bluff
Robert A. Burkich, MD
4480 Highway 70 E.
P.O. Box 185
White Bluff, TN 37187
(615) 797-3646 FAX (615) 797-4055

TEXAS
Amarillo
George Cole, DO
2300 Bell Street, #20
Amarillo, TX 79106
(806) 379-7770 FAX (806) 352-6599

Gerald Parker, DO
4714 S. Western
Amarillo, TX 79109
(806) 355-8263 FAX (806) 355-8796

John T. Taylor, DO
4714 S. Western
Amarillo, TX 79109
(806) 355-8263 FAX (806) 355-8796

Arlington
R. E. Liverman, DO
801 W. Road to Six Flags, #147
Arlington, TX 76012
(817) 461-7774 FAX (817) 801-5600

Austin
Ted Edwards Jr, MD
4201 Bee Caves Rd., #B-112
Austin, TX 78746
(512) 327-4886

Vladimir Rizov, MD
911 W. Anderson Lane, #205

Austin, TX 78757
(512) 451-8149 FAX (512) 451-0895

Conroe
Frank O. McGehee Jr, MD
900 West Davis
Conroe, TX 77301
(936) 756-3366

Euless
Marina Johnson, MD
350 Westpark Way, #120
Euless, TX 76040
(817) 358-0663 FAX (817) 358-9163

Fort Worth
Barry L. Beaty, DO
4455 Camp Bowie, #211
Fort Worth, TX 76107
(817) 737-6464 FAX (817) 737-2858

Karen Birdy, DO
1307 Eighth Ave., #206
Fort Worth, TX 76104
(817) 924-5087 FAX (817) 924-0167

Gerald Harris, DO
1550 W. Rosedale St., #714
Fort Worth, TX 76104-7411
(817) 732-2878 FAX (817) 732-9315

Joseph F. McWherter, MD
1307 - 8th Ave.,#207
Fort Worth, TX 76104
(817) 926-2511 FAX (817) 924-0167

Ricardo Tan, MD
3220 North Freeway, #106
Fort Worth, TX 76111
(817) 626-1993

Michael Truman, DO
2401 Canton Drive
Fort Worth, TX 76112
(817) 446-5500 FAX (817) 446-5509

Grapevine
Constantine A. Kotsanis, MD
1600 W. College St., #260
Grapevine, TX 76051
(817) 481-6342 FAX (817) 488-8903

Harlingen
Robert R. Somerville, MD
720 N. 77 Sunshine Strip
Harlingen, TX 78550
(956) 428-0757 FAX (956) 428-8560

Houston
Robert Battle, MD
9910 Long Point
Houston, TX 77055
(713) 932-0552 FAX (713) 932-0551

Moe Kakvan, MD
2909 Hillcroft, Ste. 250B
Houston, TX 77057
(713) 780-7019 FAX (713) 780-9783

Steven J. Levy, DO
1140 Westmont, #300
Houston, TX 77015
(713) 451-4100 FAX (713) 451-0010

Gilbert Manso, MD
5177 Richmond Ave., #125
Houston, TX 77056
(713) 840-9355 FAX (713) 840-9468

Marina M. Pearsall, MD
4126 Southwest Freeway, #1620
Houston, TX 77027
(713) 522-4037 FAX (713)623-8007

R.G. Tannerya, MD
9627 Pagewood Lane
Houston, TX 77063
(713) 278-2111

Stephen Joel Weiss, MD
P.O. Box 91062
Houston, TX 77291
(713) 691-0737 FAX (713) 695-0105

Huntsville
Frank O. McGehee Jr, MD
1909 - 22nd Street
Huntsville, TX 77340
(936) 291-3351 FAX (936) 291-3519

Irving
Frances J. Rose, MD
1701 W. Walnut Hill, #200
Irving, TX 75038
(972) 594-1111 FAX (972) 518-1867

Jefferson
Donald Ray Whitaker, DO
210 E. Elizabeth St.
Jefferson, TX 75657
(903) 665-7781 FAX (903) 665-7887

Katy
David Sheridan, MD
20214 Braidwood, #215
Katy, TX 77450
(281) 579-3600 FAX (281) 579-3698

Kirbyville
John L. Sessions, DO
1609 South Margaret
Kirbyville, TX 75956
(409) 423-2166

Lewisville
Smart Idemudia, MD
560 W. Main Street, #205
Lewisville, TX 75057
(972) 420-6777 FAX (972-420-0656

Longview
Patricia F. Sanders, MD
472 East Loop 281, Ste. B
Longview, TX 75605
(903) 236-0033 FAX (903) 234-1437

McAllen
Michael R. Kilgore, MD
3600 N. 23rd, #201
McAllen, TX 78501
(210) 687-6196

Pleasanton
Gerald Phillips, MD
218 W. Goodwin Street
Pleasanton, TX 78064
(210) 569-2118 FAX (210) 569-5958

Rowlett
Robert J. Gilbard, MD
5429 Lakeview Pkwy
Rowlett, TX 75088
(972) 463-1744 FAX (972) 463-8243

San Angelo
Benjamin Thurman, MD
610 S. Abe Street, #A
San Angelo, TX 76903
(915) 481-0596 FAX (915) 481-0597

Texas City
Dorothy Merritt, MD
1125 N. Highway 3, #100A
Texas City, TX 77591
(409) 938-1770 FAX (409) 938-0701

Victoria
Rolando G. Arafiles Jr, MD
202 James Coleman Dr., #4
Victoria, TX 77904
(361) 570-3641 FAX (361) 570-3644

Waco
William P. Coleman, MD
504 Meadow Lake Ctr.
Waco, TX 76712
(254) 776-7444 FAX (254) 776-9729

Wichita Falls
Thomas Roger Humphrey, MD
2400 Rushing
Wichita Falls, TX 76308
(940) 766-4329 FAX (940) 767-3227

UTAH
Alpine
Dianne Farley-Jones, MD
70 E. Red Pine Drive
Alpine, UT 84004
(801) 756-9444 FAX (801) 763-1070

Draper
Dennis Harper, DO
12226 S. 1000 East, #10
Draper, UT 84020
(801) 277-5000 FAX (801) 277-5200

Provo
Dennis Remington, MD
1675 N. Freedom Blvd., Suite 11E
Provo, UT 84604
(801) 373-8500 FAX (801) 373-3426

W. David Voss, DO
1675 Freedom Blvd., #11-E
Provo, UT 84604
(801) 373-8500

VERMONT
Colchester
Charles Anderson, MD
Health & Longevity Institute,
Creek Farm Plaza
65 Creek Farm Road #7
Colchester, VT 05446
(802) 879-6544

VIRGINIA
Chesapeake
Ernest Aubrey Murden Jr, MD
4020 Raintree Rd., #C
Chesapeake, VA 23321
(757) 488-2080 FAX (757) 405-3025

Falls Church
Aldo M. Rosemblat, MD
6316 Castle Place, #200
Falls Church, VA 22044
(703) 241-8989 FAX (703) 532-6247

Hinton
Harold Huffman, MD
P. O. Box 197
Hinton, VA 22831
(540) 867-5154

Louisa
David G. Schwartz, MD
P. O. Box 532
Louisa, VA 23093
(540) 967-2050

Markham
James B. Hutt, Jr., MD
2876 Leeds Manor Road
Markham, VA 22643
(540) 347-0474

McLean
Manjit R. Bajwa, MD
1007 Heather Hill Court

McLean, VA 22101
(703) 848-0807

Nellysford
Mitchell A. Fleisher, MD
P.O. Box 303
Rockfish Ctr., Suite One, SR 664
Nellysford, VA 22958
(804) 361-1896 FAX (804) 361-1928

Richmond
Peter C. Gent, DO
2621 Promenade Pkwy.
Richmond, VA 23113
(804) 897-8566 FAX (804) 897-8569

Roanoke
Joan M. Resk, DO
5249 Clearbrook Lane
Roanoke, VA 24014
(540) 776-8331 FAX (540) 776-8303

Trout Dale
Eduardo Castro, MD
799 Ripshin Road, P.O. Box 44
Trout Dale, VA 24378
(540) 677-3631 FAX (540) 677-3843

Elmer M. Cranton, MD
799 Ripshin Road, Box 44
Trout Dale, VA 24378
(540) 677-3631 FAX (540) 677-3843

WASHINGTON
Bellevue
David Buscher, MD
1603 - 116th N.E., Ste. 112
Bellevue, WA 98004-3825
(425) 453-0288 FAX (425) 455-0076

Betty Sy Go, MD
15611 Bel-Red Road
Bellevue, WA 98008
(425) 881-2224 FAX (425) 881-2216

Bellingham
Andrew Pauli, MD
1116 Key Street, #200
Bellingham, WA 98225
(360) 527-9785 FAX (360) 671-0981

Elk
Stanley B. Covert, MD
42207 N. Sylvan Road
Elk, WA 99009
(509) 292-2748

Federal Way
Thomas A. Dorman, MD
2505 South 320th St., #100
Federal Way, WA 98003
(253) 529-3050 FAX (253) 529-3104

George Koss, DO
1014 South 320th Street
Federal Way, WA 98003
(253) 839-4100 FAX (253) 941-6116

Kirkland
Jonathan Collin, MD
12911 120th Ave. NE, #A-50,
POB 8099
Kirkland, WA 98034
(425) 820-0547 FAX (425) 820-0259

Port Townsend
Jonathan Collin, MD
911 Tyler Street
Port Townsend, WA 98368
(360) 385-4555 FAX (360) 385-0699

J. Douwe Rienstra, MD
242 Monroe Street
Port Townsend, WA 98368
(360) 385-5658 FAX (360) 385-5142

Renton
Jonathan Wright, MD
801 SW 16th Street, #121
Renton, WA 98055
(425) 264-0059 FAX (425) 264-0071

Richland
Geoffrey S. Ames, MD
750 Swift Blvd., #1
Richland, WA 99397
(509) 943-3934

Seattle
Ralph Golan, MD
7522 - 20th Ave., NE

Seattle, WA 98115
(206) 524-8966 FAX (206) 524-8951

Spokane
William Corell, MD
3424 Grand Blvd. South
Spokane, WA 99203
(509) 838-5800 FAX (509) 838-4042

Burton B. Hart, DO
12104 E. Main Street
Spokane, WA 99206
(509) 927-9922 FAX (509) 926-2011

Vancouver
Steve Kennedy, MD
615 S.E. Chkalov, #14
Vancouver, WA 98683
(360) 256-4566 FAX (360) 253-3060

Winlock
David Ellis, MD
P.O. Box 567
Winlock, WA 98596
(360) 785-0300 FAX (360) 785-3330

Yelm
Elmer M. Cranton, MD
503 First Street So., #1
Yelm, WA 98597
(360) 458-1061 FAX (360) 458-1661

Stephen Olmstead, MD
503 First St. South, #1
Yelm, WA 98597
(360) 458-1061 FAX (360) 458-1661

WEST VIRGINIA
Charleston
Steve M. Zekan, MD
1208 Kanawha Blvd. E.
Charleston, WV 25301
(304) 343-7559 FAX (304) 343-1219

Hurricane
John P. MacCallum, MD
3855 Teays Valley Road
Hurricane, WV 25526
(304) 757-3368 FAX (304) 757-2402

Dallas B. Martin, DO
1401 Hospital Dr., #302
Hurricane, WV 25526
(304) 757-8090 FAX (304) 757-8079

Morgantown
Thomas Wilshire, DO
3496 University Ave.
Morgantown, WV 26505
(304) 599-7900 FAX (304) 599-6050

WISCONSIN
Delafield
Carol Uebelacker, MD
700 Milwaukee St.
Delafield, WI 53018
(262) 646-4600 FAX (262) 646-4215

Green Bay
Eleazar M. Kadile, MD
1538 Bellevue St.
Green Bay, WI 54311
(920) 468-9442 FAX (920) 468-9714

La Crosse
Patrick J. Scott, MD
3454 Losey Blvd. South.
La Crosse, WI 54601
(608) 785-0038 FAX (608) 782-5959

Milwaukee
J. Allan Robertson Jr., DO
1011 N. Mayfair Rd., #301

Milwaukee, WI 53226
(414) 302-1011 FAX (414) 302-1010

Carol Uebelacker, MD
5404-A North Lovers Lane Rd.
Milwaukee, WI 53225
(414) 466-2002 FAX (414) 466-2855

Wauwatosa
Jerry N. Yee, DO
11803 W. North Avenue
Wauwatosa, WI 53226
(414) 258-6282

Wisconsin Dells
Robert S. Waters, MD
Race & Vine Streets, Box 357
Wisconsin Dells, WI 53965
(608) 254-7178; (800) 200-7178 FAX
(608) 253-7139

WYOMING
Casper
Dennis Wicks, MD
802 South Durbin St.
Casper, WY 82601
(307) 237-4444

Gillette
Rebecca Painter, MD
201 West Lakeway, #300
Gillette, WY 82718
(307) 682-0330 FAX (307) 686-8118

Reprinted with permission from the 2001 Membership Roster of the American College for Advancement in Medicine.

NOTES

Introduction

1. Langgaard, H.; Launso, L.; Haugaard, C. "Main themes in research on unconventional cancer treatment." *Townsend Letter for Doctors and Patients*. 217/218:57–66, August/September 2001.
2. Moss, R.W. "The war on cancer." *Townsend Letter for Doctors and Patients*. 217/218:20–22, August/September 2001.
3. Richardson, M.D.; Sanders, T.; Palmer, J.L.; et al. "Complementary/alternative medicine used in a comprehensive cancer center and the implications for oncology." *Journal of Clinical Oncology*. 18(13):2502–2514, July 2000.
4. Sparber, A.; Jonas, W.; White, J.; et al. "Cancer clinical trials and subject use of natural herbal products." *Cancer Investigation*. 18(5):436–439, 2000.
5. "Mistletoe therapy found to be effective for treatment of cancer." *Townsend Letter for Doctors and Patients*. 217/218:26, August/September 2001.

Chapter 1

1. Dollinger, M.; Rosenbaum, E.H.; Cable, G. *Everyone's Guide to Cancer Therapy*. Kansas City, Kansas: Andrews McMeel Publishing, 1997, p. 10.
2. Sporn, M.B., and Roberts, A.B. "Peptide growth factors and inflammation, tissue repair and cancer." *Journal of Clinical Investigation*. 78:329–332, 1986.
3. Sporn, M.B., and Roberts, A.B. "Peptide growth factors are multifunctional." *Nature*. 332:217–219.
4. Berressem, P.; Frech, S.; Hartleb, M. "Additional therapy with Polyerga® improves immune reactivity and quality of life in breast

cancer patients during rehabilitation." *Tumor Diagnosis and Therapy.* 16:45–48, 1995.

5. Ibid.

6. Van't Veen, A.; de Ruyter, H.; Mouton, J.W.; Hartleb, M.; Lachmann, B. "Pretreatment with spleen peptides can enhance survival in influenza A infected mice." *Forsch. Komplementaermedizin* 3:218–221, 1996.

7. Vassilev, M.; Zacharieva, E.; Antonov, K.; Krastev, T. "Treatment of chronic hepatitis B patients with Polyerga®." *Journal of Hepatology.* 23 (supplement 1):197, 1995.

8. Borghardt, E.J.; Rosien, B.; Frech, S.; Harleb, M. "Polyerga® as supportive therapy could improve quality of life in head and neck cancer patients during chemotherapy." *Supportive Care in Cancer.* 3(5):96, September 1995.

9. Jurin, M.; Zarkovic, N.; Ilic, Z.; Borovic, S.; Hartleb, M. "Porcine splenic peptides (Polyerga®) decrease the number of experimental lung metastases in mice." *Clinical and Experimental Metastasis.* 14:55–60, 1996.

10. Jurin, M.; Zarkovic, N.; Borovic, S.; Hartleb, M. "Chemotherapy and spleen peptides preparation, SP-1, (Polyerga®) in the treatment of experimental lung metastases of mammary carcinoma in mice." *Croatian Medical Journal.* 38(4):317–321, 1997.

11. Zarkovic, N.; Hartleb, M.; Zarkovic, K.; Borovic, S.; Golubic, J.; Kalisnik, T.; Frech, S.; Klingmuller, M.; Loncaric, I.; Bosnjak, B.; Jurin, M.; Kuhlmey, J. "Spleen peptides (Polyerga®) inhibit development of artificial lung metastases of murine mammary carcinoma and increase efficiency of chemotherapy in mice." *Cancer Biotherapy & Radiopharmaceuticals.* 13(1):25–32, 1998.

12. Vassilev, M.; Antonov, K.; Theocharov, P.; Krastev, Z. "The effect of low molecular weight glycoproteins in chronic hepatitis B." *Hepato-Gastroenterology.* 43:882–886, 1996.

13. Chiarotto, J.; Thirmall, M.; Trudeau, M.; Skelton, J.; Boos, G.; Viallet, J. "Phase I-II trial of an unconventional agent, Polyerga®, in patients with advanced cancer." *Weekly Cancer Researcher.* March 7, 1994.

14. De Ojeda, G.; Diez-Orejas, R.; Portoles, P.; Ronda, M.; Del Pozo, M.L.; Feito, M.J.; Hartleb, M.; Rojo, J.M. "Polyerga®, a biological response modifier enhancing T-lymphocyte-dependent responses." *Research and Experimental Medicine.* 194:261–276, 1994.

15. Dollinger, M.; Rosenbaum, E.H.; Cable, G. *Everyone's Guide to Cancer Therapy: How Cancer Is Diagnosed, Treated, and Managed Day to Day.* Revised Third Edition. Kansas City, Kansas: Andrews McMeel Publishing, 1997, pp. 70–73.

16. Diamond, W.J.; Cowden, W.L.; Goldberg, B. *An Alternative Medicine Definitive Guide to Cancer.* Tiburon, California: Future Medicine Publishing, 1997, pp. 70 and 72.

17. Ibid., pp. 809–935.

18. Baier, J.E.; Neumann, H.A.; Taufighi-Chirazi, T.; Gallati, H.; Ricken, D. "Thymopentin, Factor AF2, and Polyerga® improve impaired mitogen induced interferon-g release of peripheral blood mononuclear cells derived from tumor patients." *Tumor Diagnostik & Therapie.* 1(15):21–26, February 1994.

19. Hartleb, M., and Leuschner, J. "Toxological profile of a low molecular weight spleen peptide formulation used in supportive cancer therapy." *Arznein Forschung/Drug Research.* 47(11):1047–1051, 1997.

20. Klose, G., and Mertens, J. "Long term results of post-operative treatment of carcinoma of the stomach with Polyerga®." *Therapiewoche.* 27:5359–5361, 1977.

21. Dollinger et al., 1997, pp. 430–449.

Chapter 2

1. Maar, K. "Patient K, recurrent rectal carcinoma." *Complementary Oncology Forum & Immunobiology Forum.* 2:32, May 1999.

2. Wehner, H.; Von Ardenne, A.; Kaltofen, S. "Whole-body hyperthermia with water-filtered infrared radiation: technical-physical aspects and clinical experiences." *International Journal of Hyperthermia.* 17(1):19–30, 2001.

3. *Encyclopedia Americana, International Edition.* New York: Americana Corporation, 196, 28:347.

4. Von Ardenne, M. "Principles and concept 1993 of the systemic Cancer Multistep Therapy (sCMT). Extreme whole-body hyperthermia using the infrared-A technique IRATHERM 2000—selective thermosensitization by hyperglycemia—circulatory backup by adapted hyperoxemia." *Strahlentherapie und Onkologie.* 10:581–589, 1994.

5. Von Ardenne, M. "Syncarcinolysis in Gestalt der Mehrschritt-Therapie." Vortrag in *Heidelberger Krebsforschungszentrum* 25:9, 1965.

6. Mayer, W.K.; Steinhausen, D.; Goebel, A.; Von Ardenne, M. "Acute systemic tolerance of 42.0°C infrared whole body hyperthermia in combination with hyperglycemia and hyperoxia." Poster und Vortrag, 6th International Congress on Hyperthermic Oncology. 26.4–1.5.1992, Tucson, Arizona.

7. Von Ardenne, M: Reitnauer, P.G. "Erythrozyten versteifen nicht bei Passage uebersauerter Tumoren." *Deutsche Z. Onkologie* 24:46–51, 1992.

8. Von Ardenne, M. "Die Mehrfachnutzung der einzelnen im Konzept

der Krebs-Mehrschritt-Therapie vereinigten Schritte." *Arztezeitschrift Forschung Naturheilverfahren* 31(12):955–964, 1990.

9. Hecht, H.-Ch.: Obst, H.; Schuhmann, E. "IRA-Therm II—ein Geratesystem zur Infrarot-A-Hyperthermie." Poster 6. Treffpunkt Medizintechnik 15.–16.11.1990 FU Berlin, Tagungsband S. 115.

Chapter 3

1. Moss, R.W. *The Cancer Industry.* New York: Paragon House, 1989, p. 75.
2. Glassman, J. *The Cancer Survivors.* New York: Dial Press, 1983, p. 46.
3. Moss, 1989, p. 77.
4. Diamond, W.J.; Cowden, W.L.; Goldberg, B. *An Alternative Medicine Definitive Guide to Cancer.* Tiburon, California: Future Medicine Publishing, 1997, p. 33.

Chapter 4

1. Schmidt, K.P. "Darwin, Charles Robert." *Encyclopedia Americana, International Edition.* New York: Americana Corporation, 1966, 8:485 and 486.
2. Platt, R. "Venus' Flytrap." *Encyclopedia Americana, International Edition.* New York: Americana Corporation, 1966, 28:12.
3. Lapedes, D.N. *McGraw-Hill Dictionary of Scientific and Technical Terms.* Second Edition. New York: McGraw-Hill Book Co., 1978, p. 1068.
4. Keller, H. *Carnivora® Immunomodulator & Cytostatic.* Nordhalben, Germany: Carnivora-Forschungs GmbH, 1994, pp. 1, 3, and 5.
5. Kreher, B. "Chemische und immunologische Untersuchungen der Drogen *Dionaea muscipula, Tabebuia avellanedae, Euphorbia resinifera* und *Daphne mezereum* sowie ihrer Praeparate." Dissertation. Munich: Ludwig-Maximiliansp Universitaet, 1989.
6. Kreher, B.; Neszmelyi, A.; Polos, K.; Wagner, H. "Structure elucidation of plumbagin analogs from *Dionaea muscipula* and their *in vitro* immunological activity on human granulocytes and lymphocytes." *Planta Medicina.* 55(1):112, 1989.
7. Kreher, B.; Neszmelyi, A.; Polos, K.; Wagner, H. "Structure elucidation of plumbagin-analogues from *Dionaea muscipula* and their immunomodulating activities *in vitro* and *in vivo*." *Molecular Recognition, International Symposium.* Sopron, Hungary, August 24–27, 1988. Nordhalben, Germany: Carnivora-Forschungs GmbH, 1988, p. 16.
8. Nikolov, R. personal correspondence.
9. *Carnivora: A Novel Phytopharmacon.* Nordhalben, Germany: Carnivora-Forschungs GmbH, 1992, p. 34.

Chapter 6
1. Pekar, R. *Percutaneous Bio-Electrotherapy of Cancerous Tumours: A Documentation of Basic Principles and Experiences with Bio-Electrotherapy.* Vienna, Munich, Berne: Verlag Wilhelm Maudrich, 1997.

Chapter 7
1. Moffat, F.L., et al. "Hyperthermia for cancer: a practical perspective." *Seminars in Surgical Oncology.* 1:200–219, 1985.
2. *The Merck Manual of Diagnosis and Therapy.* Rahway, New Jersey: Merck Research Laboratories, 1992, p. 2417.
3. Coley, W.B. "Late results of the treatment of inoperable sarcoma by the mixed toxins Erysipelas and *Bacillus prodigiosus.*" *American Journal of Science.* 131:375–388, 1906.
4. Selawry, O.; Goldstein, M.; McCormick, T. "Hyperthermia in tissue-cultured cells of malignant origin." *Cancer Research.* 17:785–791, 1957.
5. Crile, Jr., G. "Heat as an adjunct to the treatment of cancer." *Experimental Studies, Cleveland Clinic Quarterly.* 28:75–89, 1961.
6. Crile, Jr., G. "Selective destruction of cancers after exposure to heat." *Annals of Surgery.* 156:404–407, 1962.
7. Marmor, J.B., and Hahn, G.M. "Tumor cure and cell survival after localized radiofrequency heating." *Cancer Research.* 37:879–883, 1977.
8. Dickson, J.A., and Shah, S.A. "Immunologic aspects of hyperthermia." In: *Hyperthermia in Cancer Therapy.* Storm, F.K. (ed.). Boston: G.K. Hall Medical Publishers, 1983, pp. 487–543.
9. Marmor, J.B. "Interaction of hyperthermia and drugs in animals." *Cancer Research.* 38:2304, 1979.
10. Robinson, J.E., and Wizenberg, M.J. "Thermal sensitivity and the effect of elevated temperature on the radiation sensitivity of Chinese hamster cells." *Journal of Radiological Therapy.* (Stockholm). 13:241–248, 1974.
11. Overgard, K. "Ueber Warmtherapie boesartiger Tumoren." *Acta Radiolo. Therap.* (Stockholm). 15:89–100, 1934.
12. Warren, S.L. "Preliminary study of the effect of artificial fever upon hopeless tumor cases." *American Journal of Roentgenology.* 33:75, 1935.
13. Robinson, J.E. "Hyperthermia and oxygen enhancement ratio." In: *Proceedings of the International Symposium on Cancer Therapy, Hyperthermia and Radiation.* Washington, D.C.: American Cancer Society, 1976, pp. 66–74.
14. Mendecki, J.; Friedenthal, E.; Davis, L.W. "Hyperthermia in cancer therapy." *Einstein Quarterly Journal of Biology and Medicine,* 4:167–175, 1986.
15. Crile, 1961.

16. Crile, 1962.
17. Mendecki, J.; Friedenthal, E.; Botstein, C. "Effects of microwave-induced local hyperthermia on mammary adenocarcinoma in C3H mice." *Cancer Research.* 36:2113–2114, 1976.
18. Dickson and Shah, 1983.
19. Dewey, W.C.; Freeman, M.L.; Raaporst, G.P.; Clark, E.P.; Wong, R.S.; Highfield, D.P.; Spiro, J.S.; Tomasovic, S.P.; Denman, D.L.; Cross, R.A. "Cell biology of hyperthermia and radiation." In: *Radiation Biology in Cancer Research.* New York: Raven Press, 1980, pp. 589–623.
20. Overgaard, J. "Influence of extracellular pH on the viability and morphology of tumor cells exposed to hyperthermia." *Journal of the National Cancer Institute.* 56:12453–1250, 1976.
21. Song, C.W. "Effect of local hyperthermia on blood flow and microenvironment: a review." *Cancer Research* (supplement). 44:4721–4730, 1984.
22. Henle, K.J., and Dethlefsen, L.A. "Heat fractionation and thermotolerance: a review." *Cancer Research.* 38:1843–1851, 1978.
23. Strauss, A.A.; Appel, M.; Saphir, O.; Rabinowitz, A.J. "Immunologic resistance to carcinoma produced by electrocoagulation." *Surgical Gynecology and Obstetrics.* 121:989–996, 1965.
24. Stehlin, J.S. "Hyperthermic perfusion of the extremities for melanomas and sarcomas." *American Journal of Roentgenology, Radium Therapy, and Nuclear Medicine.* 130:191–196, 1978.
25. Sugaar, S., and Leveen, H.H. "A histopathologic study on the effects of radiofrequency thermotherapy on malignant tumors of the lung." *Cancer,* 43:767–783, 1979.

Chapter 8

1. Hirazumi, A.; Furusawa, E.; Chou, S.C.; Hokama, Y. "Anticancer activity of *Morinda citrifolia* (noni) on intraperitoneally implanted Lewis lung carcinoma in syneneic mice." *Proceedings of the Western Pharmacological Society.* 37:145–146, 1994.
2. Hirazumi, A.; Furusawa, E.; Chou, S.C.; Hokama, Y. "Immunomodulation contributes to the anticancer activity of *Morinda citrifolia* (noni) fruit juice." *Proceedings of the Western Pharmacological Society.* 39:25–27, 1996.
3. Levand, O., and Larson, H. "Some chemical constituents of *Morinda citrifolia.*" *Planta Medica.* 36:186–187, 1979.
4. Wang, M.; Kikuzaki, H.; Csiszar, K.; Boyd, C.D.; Maunakes, A.; Fong, S.F.T.; Ghai, G.; Rosen, R.T.; Nakatani, N.; Ho, C.-T. "Novel trisaccharide fatty acid ester identified from the fruits of *Morinda citrifolia* (noni)." *Journal of Agriculture and Food Chemistry.* 47:4880–4882, 1999.
5. Kaltsas, H. "Prescribe for yourself: how to make alternative medicine

work for you. Noni: from legend to promising nutriceutical."*Alternative Medicine* 39: 70–75, January 2001.

6. Ibid.

7. Younos, C.; Rolland, A.; Fleurentin, J.; Lanchers, M.C.; Misslin, R.; Mortier, F. "Analgesic and behavioral effects of *Morinda citrifolia*." *Planta Medica*. 56:430–434, 1990.

8. Heinicke, R.M. "The pharmacologically active ingredient of noni." *Bulletin of the Pacific Tropical Botanical Garden*. 15:1014, 1985.

9. Daulatabad, C.D.; Mulia, G.M.; Mirajkar, A.M. "Ricinoleic acid in *Morinda citrifolia* seed oil." *Journal of the Oil Technology Association* (India). 21:26–27, 1989.

10. Rusia, K., and Srivastava, S.K. "A new anthraquinones from the roots of *Morinda citrifolia*." *Current Science*. 58:249, 1989.

11. Jain, R.K., Ravindra, K.; Srivastava, S.D. "Two new anthraquinones in the roots of *Morinda citrifolia*." *Proceedings of the National Science Institute of India, Section A*. 62:11–13, 1992.

12. Srivastrava, M., and Singh, J. "A new anthraquinone glycoside from *Morinda citrifolia*." *International Journal of Pharmacognosy*. 58:249, 1989.

13. Tiwari, R.D., and Singh, J. "Structural study of the anthraquinone glycosides from the flowers of *Morinda citrifolia*." *Journal of the Indian Chemical Society*. 54:429–430, 1977.

14. Singh, J., and Tiwari, R.D. "Flavone glycosides from the flowers of *Morinda citrifolia*." *Journal of the Indian Chemical Society*. 58:424, 1976.

Chapter 9

1. Ohno, R.; Imai, K.; Yokomaku, S.; Yamada, K. "Antitumor effect of protein-bound polysaccharide preparation, PS-K, against the 3-methylcholanthrene-induced fibrosarcoma in C57BL/6 mice." *Gann* (Japan). 66:679–681, 1975.

2. Arora, D. *All That the Rain Promises and More*. Berkeley, California: Ten Speed Press, 1991.

3. Gilbertson, R.L., and Ryvarden, L. *North American Polypores*. Oslo, Norway: Fungiflora, 1986.

4. Arora, D. *Mushrooms Demystified*. Berkeley, California: Ten Speed Press, 1986.

5. Namba, T.K. *Genshoku Wakanyaku Zukan*. Osaka, Japan: Hoikusha, 1980, p. 247.

6. Yang, Q.Y., et al. "A new biological response modifier—PSP." In: *Mushroom Biology and Mushroom Products*. S.-T. Chang et al. (eds.). Hong Kong: Chinese University Press, 1993, pp. 247–259.

7. Hobbs, C. *Medicinal Mushrooms: An Exploration of Tradition, Healing, and Culture*. Third Edition. Loveland, Colorado: Interweave Press, December 1996, p. 161.

8. Sakagami, H., and Takeda, M. "Diverse biological activity of PSK (Krestin), a protein-bound polysaccharide from *Coriolus versicolor.*" *Proceedings of the First International Conference on Mushroom Biology and Mushroom Products.* August 23–26, 1993, Chinese University of Hong Kong, Hong Kong.

9. *Mushroom Biology and Mushroom Products.* Chang, S.-T., et al. (eds.). Shatin, Hong Kong: Chinese University Press, 1993, pp. 237–245.

10. Yang et al., 1993.

11. Itoh, I.; Sakai, T.; Mori, T. "Aspects of immunological antitumor agent and its clinical use of PSK." *Japanese Journal of Cancer Chemotherapy.* 6:681, 1994.

12. Kumashiro, R.; Hiramoto, Y.; Okamura, T.; Kano, T.; Sano, C.C.; Inokuchi, K. "Postoperative long-term immunostimulatory protein-bound polysaccharide Kureha (PSK) therapy for advanced gastric cancer." In: Torisu, M.; Yoshida, T. (eds.). *Basic Mechanisms and Clinical Treatment of Tumor Metastasis.* New York: Academic Press, 1985, p. 523.

13. Mitomi, T., and Ogoshi, K. "Clinical study of PSK as an adjuvant immunochemotherapeutic agent against gastric cancer." *Japanese Journal of Cancer Chemotherapy.* 13:2532, 1992.

14. Nakazato, H.; Ichihashi, H.; Kondo, T. "Clinical results of a randomized controlled trial on the effect of adjuvant immunochemotherapy using Esquinon and Krestin for patients with curatively resected gastric cancer." *Japanese Journal of Cancer Chemotherapy.* 13:308, 1993.

15. Nimoto, M.; Toge, T.; Nakano, A.; Yanagawa, E.; Oride, M.; Hirano, M.; Nakanishi, K.; Nosou, Y.; Yamada, Y.; Hattori, T. "Adjuvant immunochemotherapy in patients with gastric cancer." *Japanese Journal of Gastroenterological Surgery.* 14:704, 1990.

16. Shiraki, S.; Mori, H.; Ito, A.; Kadomoto, N.; Yamagiwa, S.; Yamada, Y.; Noda, K. "Adjuvant immunotherapy for carcinoma of uterine cervix with PSK." *Japanese Journal of Cancer Chemotherapy.* 9:1031, 1994.

17. Ikeda, T.; Sakai, T.; Saito, T.; Kosaki, G. "Evaluation of postoperative immunochemotherapy for lung cancer patients." *Japanese Journal of Cancer Chemotherapy.* 13:1044, 1991.

18. Torisu, M.; Hayashi, Y.; Ishimitsu, T.; Fujimura, T.; Iwasaki, K.; Katano, M.; Yamamoto, H.; Kimura, Y.; Takesue, M.; Kondo, M.; Nomoto, K. "Significant prolongation of disease-free period gained by oral polysaccharide K (PSK) administration after curative surgical operation of colorectal cancer." *Cancer Immunology & Immunotherapy.* 31:261–268, 1990.

19. Itoro, S. "Enhancement of antitumor cell toxicity for hepatic lymphocytes by oral administration of PSK." *International Journal of Immunopharmacology.* 16(2):123–130, 1994.

20. Etoe, K. "Activation of human natural killer cells by the protein-

bound polysaccharide PSK independently of interferon and inter-leucin II." *Immunology Letters.* 31:241–246, 1992.

21. Ebihara, M. "Peptide effect of biological response modifiers on murine cytomegalovirus infection." *Journal of Virology.* 51(1):117–122, July 1984.

22. Zhu, D. "Recent advances on the active components in Chinese medicines." *Abstracts of Chinese Medicines.* 1:251–286, 1987.

23. Mayer, P., and Drews, J. "The effect of a protein-bound polysaccharide from *Coriolus versicolor* on immunological parameters and experimental infections in mice." *Infection.* 8:13–21, 1980.

24. Nomoto, K., et al. "Restoration of antibody-forming capacities by PS-K in tumor-bearing mice." *Gann.* 66:365–374, 1975.

25. Tsukagoshi, S., et al. "Krestin (PSK)." *Cancer Treatment Reviews.* 11:131–155, 1984.

26. Ebina, T. "Antitumor effect of PSK. (2) Effector mechanism of an-timetastatic effect in the 'double grafted tumor system'." *Gon to Kagaku Ryoho.* 14:1847–1853, 1987.

27. Tsukagoshi, 1984.

28. Tochikura, T.S., et al. "A biological response modifier, PSK, inhibits human immunodeficiency virus infection in vitro." *Biochemistry, Biophysics Research Communications.* 148:726–733, 1987.

29. Ebina, T., et al. "Antitumor effect of PSK. (1) Interferon inducing activity and intratumoral administration." *Gon to Kagaku Ryoho.* 14:1847–1853, 1987.

30. Yagashita, K., et al. "Effects of *Grifola frondosa, Coriolus versicolor,* and *Lentinus edodes* on cholesterol metabolism in rats." *Nihon Daigaku No-Juigakubo Gakujutsu Kenkyu Hokoku.* 34:1–13, 1977.

31. Liu, B., et al. "A new species of the genus *Cordyceps.*" *Journal of Wuhan Botanical Research.* 3:23–24. In: *Abstracts of Chinese Medicines.* 1:248, 1985.

32. Malone, M.H., et al. "Hippocratic screening of sixty-six species of higher fungi." *Lloydia* 30:250–257, 1967.

33. "Anticancer botanicals that work supportively with chemotherapy." *Alternative Medicine Digest.* 19:84, August/September 1997.

34. Yakawa, K.; Mitsuhashi, N.; Saito, Y.; Takahashi, M.; Katano, S.; Shiojima, K.; Furuta, M.; Niibe, H. "Effect of Krestin (PSK) as adjuvant treatment on the prognosis after radical radiotherapy in patients with non–small cell lung cancer." *Anticancer Research.* 13:1815–1820, 1993.

35. Nakazato, H.; Koike, A.; Saji, S.; Ogawa, N.; Sakamoto, J. "Efficacy of immunochemotherapy as adjuvant treatment after curative resection of gastric cancer." *Lancet.* 343:1122–1126, 1994.

36. Iino, Y.; Yokoe, T.; Maemura, M.; Horiguchi, J.; Takei, H.; Ohwada, S.;

Morishita, Y. "Immunochemotherapies versus chemotherapy as adjuvant treatment after curative resection of operable breast cancer." *Anticancer Research.* 15:2907–2912, 1995.

37. Nagao, T.; Komatsuda, M.; Yamauchi, K.; Nozaki, H.; Watanabe, K.; Arimori, S. "Chemoimmunotherapy with Krestin in acute leukemia." *Tokai Journal of Experimental Clinical Medicine.* 6(2):141–146, 1981.

Chapter 11

1. Morra, M., and Potts, E. *Choices: Realistic Alternatives in Cancer Treatment.* New York: Avon Books, 1980, pp. 50–97.

2. Bogoch, S.; Bogoch, E.S.; Faver, C.A.; Harris, J.H.; Ambrus, J.L.; Lux, W.E.; Ransohoff, J.A. "Determination of anti-malignin antibody and malignin in 1,026 cancer patients and controls: relation of antibody to survival." *Journal of Medicine.* 13:49–69, 1982.

3. Bogoch, S.; Bogoch, E.S.; Antich, P.; Dungan, S.M.; Harris, J.H.; Ambrus, J.L.; Powers, N. "Elevated levels of anti-malignin antibody quantitatively related to longer survival in cancer patients." *Protides Biological Fluids.* 31:739–747, 1984.

4. Walker, M. "The anti-malignin antibody in serum assay." *Townsend Letter for Doctors and Patients.* 107:462–464, June 1992.

INDEX